G. MATHIS K. D. LESSNAU (Eds.) **Atlas of Chest Sonography**

Springer

Berlin
Heidelberg
New York
Hong Kong
London
Milan
Paris
Tokyo

G. MATHIS   K. D. LESSNAU (Editors)

Atlas
of Chest Sonography

With Contributions by
J. T. ANNEMA, H. D. BECKER, S. BECKH, R. BITSCHNAU,
W. BLANK, C. GÖRG, F. HERTH, G. MATHIS, K. F. RABE,
J. REUSS, A. SCHULER and M. VESELIC

With 256 Figures in 447 Separate Illustrations,
Some in Color and 36 Tables

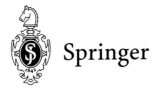

Springer

Prof. Dr. med. Gebhard Mathis
Krankenhaus der Stadt Hohenems
Interne Abteilung
Bahnhofstraße 31, 6845 Hohenems, Austria

Klaus Dieter Lessnau, MD, FCCP
Madison Medical, LLP
110 East 59th Street, Suite 9C, New York, NY10022-1304, USA

Title of the original German Edition:
G. Mathis (Hrsg.), Bildatlas der Lungen- und Pleurasonographie, 3. Auflage
© Springer-Verlag Berlin Heidelberg 2001
ISBN 3-540-67601-5

ISBN 3-540-44262-6 Springer-Verlag Berlin Heidelberg New York

Cataloging-in-Publication Data applied for

Bibliographic information published by Die Deutsche Bibliothek
Die Deutsche Bibliothek lists this publication in the Deutsche Nationalbibliografie; detailed bibliographic data
is available in the Internet at <http://dnb.ddb.de>.

Springer-Verlag Berlin Heidelberg New York
a member of BertelsmannSpringer Science+Business Media GmbH
http://www.springer.de

© Springer-Verlag Berlin Heidelberg 2003
Printed in Germany

Cover design: Frido Steinen-Broo, Pau, Spain
Typesetting: Fotosatz-Service Köhler GmbH, Würzburg, Germany
Printing and binding: Stürtz AG, Würzburg, Germany

Printed on acid-free paper   21/3150/op   5 4 3 2 1 0

Preface

The diagnostic potential of sonography in the clarification of pleural and lung diseases has long been underestimated. The ultrasound beam is fully reflected by the bony thorax and is largely obliterated by the ventilated lung. Such adverse conditions for the ultrasound beam have given rise to, and nurtured, the unjustified prejudice that sonography is of little value in this region.

Pleural effusion alone has long been a domain of ultrasonographic diagnosis. However, A-scans performed as early as the 1960s showed that peripheral lung consolidations of various origins cause a pathological transmission of the ultrasound beam, which also serves as a key to ultrasonographic imaging of peripheral lung diseases.

The past 15 years have witnessed a large number of original papers that systematically show the potential uses as well as limitations of chest sonography. After having published two monographs (1992, 1996), I considered the time ripe for a book produced by several authors, designed as a pictorial atlas, showing ultrasonography of the lung and the pleura in a compact yet comprehensive manner.

The real treasures of this book are its pictures, which encompass nearly everything that can be seen in this region. However, of equal significance is the fact that the team of authors thoroughly reviewed and exchanged their knowledge at numerous courses and state-of-the-art meetings. Thus, a critical inventory based on science and clinical practice was developed without overtaxing the method.

The subject matter of the book is primarily arranged in terms of anatomy and etiology. Two chapters focusing on the approach from clinical routine are included, namely the white hemithorax and the staged diagnostic procedure.

I sincerely thank the authors for their creative cooperation, in particular Sonja Beckh and Joachim Reuss for their ideas concerning new concepts. I am also indebted to my team who spent several years in developmental work. Otto Gehmacher gave the project a great deal of impetus. My thanks go to my family for their many-faceted support and to my daughter Lucia for her help in preparing the manuscript. Finally, I thank Sujata Wagner for translation and the staff of Springer-Verlag for their willing cooperation and careful preparation of the material.

I hope we will be able to help a large number of colleagues and serve our patients well with this pictorial atlas. Its purpose will be achieved if it helps in making diagnoses at the bedside rapidly, accurately, efficiently and economically, and also in initiating the appropriate therapy at the appropriate time.

Hohenems, January 2003   GEBHARD MATHIS

Preface

I am pleased to be co-editor for Professor Gebhard Mathis' picture atlas of lung and pleural sonography. Over the past 25 years, ultrasound equipment has improved dramatically. Multiple clinical studies have increased our knowledge to apply this technology in the daily management of patients. In the near future, hand-held point-of-care technology will spread ultrasound examinations widely among health care professionals and will supplement – and maybe even replace – the stethoscope.

Professor Mathis' book includes sections on indications, devices, techniques, yields and benefits, and complications. The reviews on pleural, pulmonary, and mediastinal diseases are excellent. The photographs are of high quality and certainly useful for the practicing pulmonologist. The figures contain the stem of the patient's history. This patient-centered approach facilitates the understanding of sensitivity and specificity of the sonographic examination. The chapter on the "wipe-out" or "white-out" lung is comprehensive and a must-read for the pulmonologist. Artifacts and pitfalls are discussed in a separate chapter. Interventional sonography is discussed and provides a useful aid to deciding on referral to a specialized center. Additional and complementary studies and techniques are addressed.

American pulmonologists may not be familiar with real-time sonography. Interestingly, with the revolutionary advent of hand-held devices (PDAs such as the Visor Prism, Handspring, and other devices) and the use of the expansion slot for a small sonogram transducer, real-time sonography will soon complement the ubiquitous use of the stethoscope. Why should the sonogram remain exclusively within the Department of Radiology if the "Department of Stethoscopology" does not even exist? The application of real-time sonography will become democratized and it will be used by many trainees and practicing pulmonologists, radiologists and internists to decrease the rate of procedure-related complications and to improve the quality of care.

In summary, this extensive review of pulmonary and pleural disease is strongly recommended for the practicing pulmonologist. I encourage pulmonologists to use this knowledge for improved and cost-effective patient care. The time is certainly well invested.

New York, January 2003   KLAUS DIETER LESSNAU

Contents

1 Indications, Technical Prerequisites, and Investigation Procedure
S. BECKH

1.1 Indications 1
1.2 Technical Requirements in Terms of Equipment 3
1.3 Investigation Procedure 3
    Summary 6
    References 6

2 The Chest Wall
R. BITSCHNAU, G. MATHIS

2.1 Soft-Tissue Lesions 7
2.2 Lymph Nodes
    (Inflammatory Lymph Nodes, Lymph Node Metastases) 9
2.3 Lesions of the Bony Chest 12
    Summary 15
    References 16

3 The Pleura
J. REUSS

3.1 Normal Pleura 17
3.2 Pleural Effusion 18
3.3 Solid Pleural Changes 22
3.4 The Diaphragm 31
    Summary 34
    References 34

4 Peripheral Lung Consolidation

4.1 Inflammatory Consolidations in the Lung: Pneumonia
    G. MATHIS 37
    Summary 48
    References 48

4.2 Neoplastic Consolidations in the Lung:
    Primary Lung Tumors and Metastases
    S. BECKH 50
    Summary 55
    References 56

4.3   Vascular Lung Consolidations:
      Pulmonary Embolism and Pulmonary Infarction
      G. Mathis 57
      Summary 70
      References 70

4.4   Mechanical Lung Consolidations: Atelectasis
      C. Görg 72
      Summary 89
      References 89

4.5   Congenital Pulmonary Sequestration
      G. Mathis 90
      References 90

5   Mediastinum

5.1   Mediastinum – Transthoracic
      W. Blank 91
      Summary 102
      References 103

5.2   Mediastinum – Transesophageal
      J. T. Annema, M. Veselic, K. F. Rabe 104
      Summary and Future Perspectives 111
      References 111

6   Endobronchial Ultrasound
      F. Herth, H. D. Becker

6.1   Instruments and Technique 113
6.2   Sonographic Anatomy 114
6.3   Results of Clinical Application 115
      Summary and Future Perspectives 117
      References 117

7   The White Hemithorax
      C. Görg

7.1   Predominantly Liquid Space-Occupying Mass 119
7.2   Predominantly Solid Space-Occupying Mass 125

8   Image Artifacts and Pitfalls
      A. Schuler

8.1   Imaging of Marginal Surfaces of the Pleura and the Diaphragm . . 138
8.2   B-Mode Artifacts 139
8.3   Color Doppler Artifacts and Pitfalls in the Thorax 143
      Summary 145
      References 145

9   Interventional Chest Sonography
W. BLANK

9.1 Ultrasound- or Computed Tomography-Guided Puncture 148
9.2 Apparatus, Instruments, and Puncture Technique 148
9.3 Indications 154
9.4 Risks 159
     Summary 160
     References 161

10   Stepwise Diagnostic Imaging Procedures in Pneumology
S. BECKH

10.1 Chest Pain 163
10.2 Pleural Disease 165
10.3 Pneumonia 167
10.4 Diffuse Pulmonary Disease 170
10.5 Pulmonary Nodule 170
10.6 Bronchial Carcinoma 173
10.7 Search for Metastases in the Lung and Pleura 175
      References 175

Subject Index 177

List of Contributors

ANNEMA, JOUKE T., Dr.
Longziekten, C3-P
Leids Universitair Medisch Centrum
Postbus 9600
2300 RC Leiden
Netherlands

BECKER, HEINRICH D., Prof. Dr.
Innere Medizin/Pulmonologie
Amalienstraße 5
69126 Heidelberg
Germany

BECKH, SONJA, OÄ Dr.
Klinikum Nürnberg Nord
Flurstraße 17
90340 Nürnberg
Germany

BITSCHNAU, ROBERT, Dr.
Innere Abteilung
Landeskrankenhaus Feldkirch
6807 Feldkirch-Tisis
Austria

BLANK, WOLFGANG, OA Dr.
Klinikum am Steinenberg,
Kreiskliniken Reutlingen,
Medizinische Klinik
Akademisches Lehrkrankenhaus
der Universität Tübingen
Steinenbergstraße 31
72764 Reutlingen
Germany

GÖRG, CHRISTIAN, Priv. Doz. Dr.
Zentrum für innere Medizin
Baldingerstraße
35043 Marburg
Germany

HERTH, FELIX, Dr.
Innere Medizin/Pulmonologie
Amalienstraße 5
69126 Heidelberg
Germany

MATHIS, GEBHARD, Prof. Dr.
Krankenhaus der Stadt Hohenems
Interne Abteilung
Bahnhofstraße 31
6845 Hohenems
Austria

RABE, K. F., Prof. Dr.
Longziekten, C3-P
Leids Universitair Medisch Centrum
Postbus 9600
2300 RC Leiden
Netherlands

REUSS, JOACHIM, OA Dr.
Medizinische Klinik
Bunsenstraße 120
71032 Böblingen
Germany

SCHULER, ANDREAS, OA Dr.
II. Medizinische Klinik, Städt. Kliniken
Am Gesundbrunnen 20
74078 Heilbronn
Germany

VESELIC, M., Dr.
Department of Pathology, C2-R
Leids Universitair Medisch Centrum
Postbus 9600
2300 RC Leiden
Netherlands

1 Indications, Technical Prerequisites, and Investigation Procedure

S. Beckh

1.1
Indications

Ultrasonography has long been established as a supplementary imaging procedure in the diagnosis of pleural effusions. Technical advancement and ongoing scientific evidence have led to the steady broadening in recent years of sonography's spectrum of application in diseases of the chest (Schwerk and Görg 1993; Stender et al. 1994; Broaddus and Light 1994; Müller 1997; Kinasewitz 1998) (Fig. 1.1).

The sonographic image does not provide a complete overview of the chest; however, it does image a certain section of it, which, given a specific problem under investigation, provides valuable additional information to substantiate overview radiographs. Occasionally, sonography is the only non-invasive diagnostic procedure that throws significant light on pathological findings (Walz and Muhr 1990; Fraser et al. 1999).

Up to 99% of ultrasound waves are reflected in the healthy lung. Intrapulmonary processes can be detected by sonography only when they extend up to the visceral pleura or can be imaged through a sound-conducting medium such as fluid or consolidated lung tissue (Fig. 1.2).

Areas of sonic shadow are caused by almost complete absorption of the ultrasound wave in bone, especially behind the sternum, scapula, and vertebral column. Any interference caused by rib shadows can be at least partially compensated with respiratory mechanics.

From a percutaneous route, the immediate retrosternal and posterior portions of the mediastinum cannot be viewed. A complementary method

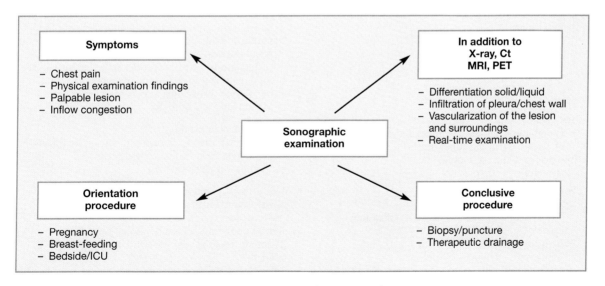

Fig. 1.1. Spectrum of application of sonography for pleural and pulmonary disease

for this location is transesophageal and transbronchial sonography which, however, are invasive investigation procedures in terms of effort and handling (Lam and Becker 1996; Arita et al. 1996; Silvestri et al. 1996; Becker 1996, 1997; Broderick et al. 1997; Serna et al. 1998; Aabakken et al. 1999) (Fig. 1.3).

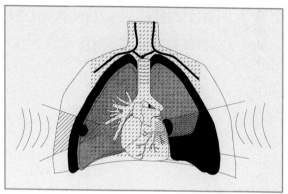

▶

Fig. 1.2. Sonographically accessible structures and pathological changes

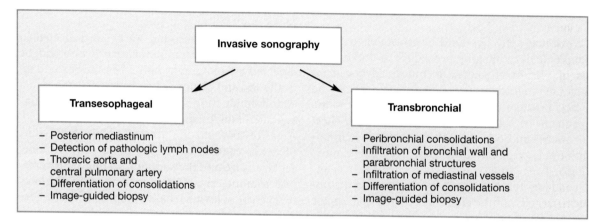

Fig. 1.3. Indications for invasive sonography

Table 1.1. Diagnostic information provided by sonography of individual thoracic structures

Thorax wall 　Benign lesions 　　Benign neoplasms (e.g., lipoma) 　　Hematoma 　　Abscess 　　Reactivated lymph nodes 　　Perichondritis, Tietze's syndrome 　　Rib fracture 　Malignant lesions 　　Lymph node metastases (initial diagnosis and course of disease during treatment) 　Invasive, growing carcinomas 　　Osteolysis **Pleura** 　Solid structures 　　Thickening of the pleura, callus, calcification, asbestosis plaques 　Space-occupying mass 　　Benign: fibrous tumor, lipoma 　　Malignant: circumscribed metastases, diffuse carcinosis, malignant pleural mesothelioma	Fluid 　Effusion, hematothorax, pyothorax, chylothorax Dynamic investigation 　Pneumothorax 　Distinguishing between effusion and callus formation 　Adherence of a space-occupying mass 　Invasion by a space-occupying mass 　Mobility of the diaphragm **Peripheral foci in the lung** 　Benign: inflammation, abscess, embolism, atelectasis 　Malignant: peripheral metastasis, peripheral carcinoma, tumor/atelectasis **Mediastinum, percutaneous** Space-occupying masses in the upper anterior mediastinum Lymph nodes in the aortopulmonary window Thrombosis of the vena cava and its supplying branches Imaging collateral circulation Pericardial effusion

Sonography provides diagnostic information when individual structures of the thorax are investigated (Table 1.1).

Further pathological alterations in the heart visualized by ultrasonography will not be described in this book. For this subject, the reader is referred to pertinent textbooks on echocardiography.

1.2
Technical Requirements in Terms of Equipment

Any equipment used for ultrasonographic investigation of the abdomen and thyroid may also be used to examine the thorax. A high-resolution linear transducer of 5–7.5 MHz is suitable for imaging the *thorax wall* and the *parietal pleura* (Mathis 1997a, b). More recently introduced probes of 10–13 MHz are excellent for evaluating *lymph nodes*. For investigating the lung, a convex or sector probe of 3–4 MHz provides adequate depth of penetration (Mathis 1997a, b).

Vector, sector, or narrow convex probes are recommended for the *mediastinum*. The smaller the connecting surface, the better the transducer can be placed in the jugular fossa or the supraclavicular fossa. The range of frequency should be 3.5–5 MHz. It should be noted that device settings commonly used for examining the heart are not suitable for the rest of the mediastinum. Contrast, image rate, and gray-scale depth balance must be adjusted to image mediastinal structures.

Transesophageal sonography requires a special probe with a suitable connecting tube to the ultrasonography device. Endobronchial sonography is performed with special, thin high-frequency probes (12–20 MHz) that are introduced via the working tube of the flexible bronchoscope. Currently, very few manufacturers offer suitable probes with an ultrasonography unit.

1.3
Investigation Procedure

The investigation is performed as far as possible with the patient seated, during inspiration and expiration, in combination with respiratory maneuvers such as coughing or „sniffing" if necessary. Raising the arms and crossing them behind the head causes intercostal spaces to be extended and facilitates

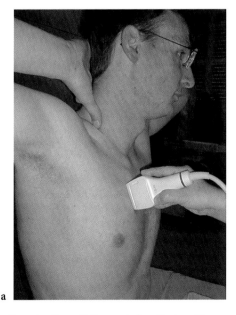
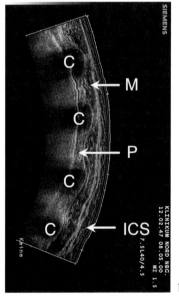

Fig. 1.4a, b. Examination of the seated patient. a Linear probe placed longitudinally on the right parasternal line. b Corresponding sonographic longitudinal panoramic image (SieScape). *C*, cartilage at the point of insertion of rib; *ICS*, intercostal space; *M*, muscle; *P*, pleural line

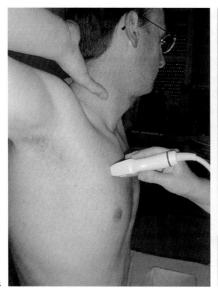
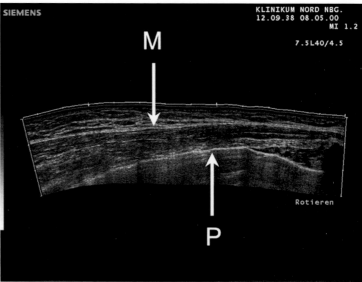

Fig. 1.5 a, b. Examination of the seated patient. a Linear probe placed parallel to the ribs in the 3rd intercostal space. b Corresponding sonographic transverse panoramic image (SieScape). *M*, muscle; *P*, pleural line

access. The transducer is moved from ventral to dorsal along the longitudinal lines in the thorax (Fig. 1.4):

- Parasternal line
- Middle and lateral clavicular line
- Anterior, middle, and posterior axillary line
- Lateral and medial scapular line
- Paravertebral line

Every finding should be allocated to its respective anatomic location and the latter should be specifically mentioned.

Subsequent transverse transducer movement parallel to the ribs in the intercostal space (Fig. 1.5) provides the additional information required for accurate localization of the respective finding.

The investigation of foci behind the scapula needs maximum adduction of the arms until the contralateral shoulder is encircled (Fig. 1.6).

Supraclavicular access allows the investigator to view the tip of the lung and the region of the brachial plexus.

Using a suprasternal approach, the anterior upper mediastinum can be viewed. The diaphragm is examined from the abdomen, in the subcostal section by the transhepatic route on the right side

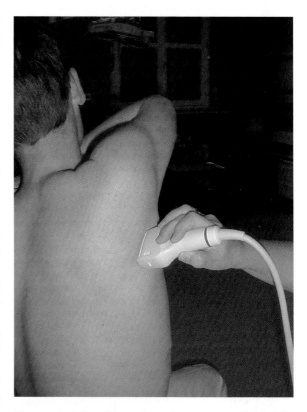

Fig. 1.6. Position of the patient when structures behind the scapula are examined

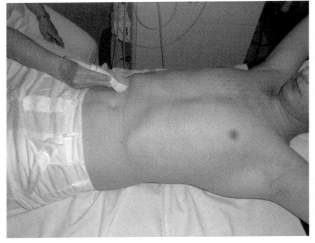
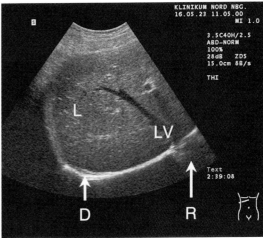

a   b

Fig. 1.7a, b. Transhepatic examination. a Convex probe placed subcostally from the right. Slight tilting in cranial direction. b Corresponding sonographic image. L, liver; LV, liver vein; D, diaphragm; R, reflection of the liver above the diaphragm

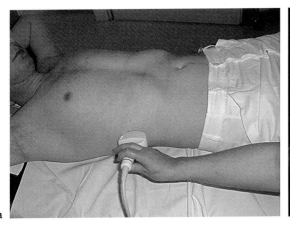
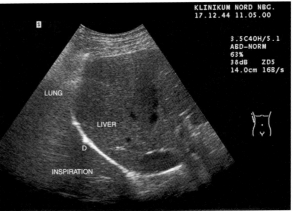

a   b

Fig. 1.8a, b. Examination from the lateral aspect. a Convex probe placed longitudinally in the mid portion of the right axillary line. b Corresponding sonographic image; D, diaphragm. The normal mobile lung is shifted during inspiration into the phrenicocostal recess and covers the upper margin of the liver

(Fig. 1.7) and, to a lesser extent, through the spleen on the left side.

Additionally, the longitudinal resonance plane from the flank images both phrenicocostal recesses (Fig. 1.8).

The supine patient is examined in the same manner. The abdominal access is better for this purpose. However, viewing intercostal spaces might be more difficult, as the mobility of the shoulder girdle is usually somewhat restricted.

The procedure for transesophageal and transbronchial sonography is described in the respective chapters.

Summary

The high resolution of the sonographic image and the real-time examination make a major contribution to the diagnosis of diseases of the chest. Structures of the chest wall and pleural lesions are visualized by ultrasound. Pulmonary consolidations are detected if they reach the visceral pleura, or if they are situated behind an acoustic window. The anterior and superior mediastinum is accessible percutaneously with certain positions of the probe. For thoracic sonography a linear probe (5–7.5 MHz) for close resolution and a convex or sector transducer (3.5–5 MHz) for access to deeper areas is recommended.

References

Aabakken L, Silvestri GA, Hawes R et al. (1999) Cost-efficacy of endoscopic ultrasonography with fine-needle aspiration vs. mediastinotomy in patients with lung cancer and suspected mediastinal adenopathy. Endoscopy 31:707–711

Arita T, Matsumoto T, Kuramitsu T et al. (1996) Is it possible to differentiate malignant mediastinal nodes from benign nodes by size? Reevaluation by CT, transesophageal echocardiography, and nodal specimen. Chest 110:1004–1008

Becker HD (1996) Endobronchialer Ultraschall – Eine neue Perspektive in der Bronchologie. Ultraschall in Med 17:106–112

Becker HD, Messerschmidt E, Schindelbeck F et al. (1997) Endobronchialer Ultraschall. Pneumologie 51:620–629

Broaddus VC, Light RW (1994) Disorders of the pleura: General principles and diagnostic approach. In: Murray JF, Nadel JA (Hrsg) Textbook of respiratory medicine. Saunders, Philadelphia, S 638–644

Broderick LS, Tarver RD, Conces DJ Jr (1997) Imaging of lung cancer: old and new. Semin Oncol 24:411–418

Fraser RS, Müller NL, Colman N, Paré PD (1999) Fraser and Paré's Diagnosis of Diseases of the Chest. Saunders, Philadelphia, S 299–338

Kinasewitz GT (1998) Disorders of the pleural space. Pleural fluid dynamics and effusions. In: Fishman AP (ed) Fishman's pulmonary diseases and disorders. McGraw-Hill, New York, S 1396–1397

Lam S, Becker HD (1996) Future diagnostic procedures. Chest Surg Clin N Am 6:363–380

Mathis G (1997a) Thoraxsonography – Part I: Chest wall and pleura. Ultrasound Med Biol 23:1131–1139

Mathis G (1997b) Thoraxsonography – Part II: Peripheral pulmonary consolidation. Ultrasound Med Biol 23:1141–1153

Müller W (1997) Ultraschall-Diagnostik. In: Rühle KH (Hrsg) Pleura-Erkrankungen. Kohlhammer, Stuttgart, S 31–44

Schwerk WB, Görg C (1993) Pleura und Lunge. In: Braun B, Günther RW, Schwerk WB (Hrsg) Ultraschalldiagnostik-Lehrbuch und Atlas. Ecomed, Landsberg, 12. Ergänzungslieferung

Serna DL, Aryan HE, Chang KJ et al. (1998) An early comparison between endoscopic ultrasound-guided fine-needle aspiration and mediastinoscopy for diagnosis of mediastinal malignancy. Am Surg 64:1014–1018

Silvestri GA, Hoffmann BJ, Bhutani MS et al. (1996) Endoscopic ultrasound with fine-needle aspiration in the diagnosis and staging of lung cancer. Ann Thorac Surg 61:1441–1445

Stender HS, Majewski A, Schober O et al. (1994) Bildgebende Verfahren in der Pneumologie. In: Ferlinz R (Hrsg) Pneumologie in Praxis und Klinik. Thieme, Stuttgart, S176–178

Walz M, Muhr G (1990) Sonographische Diagnostik beim stumpfen Thoraxtrauma. Unfallchirurg 93:359–363

2 The Chest Wall

R. BITSCHNAU, G. MATHIS

The chest wall – with the exception of the parietal pleura behind the bony ribs – can be easily visualized sonographically due to its proximity to the ultrasound (US) transducer (Sakai et al. 1990). All suspicious palpable findings in the chest wall can be an indication for chest sonography, and clinical decision-making is often based on follow-up examinations or US-guided punctures. A reliable indication for chest ultrasound is any form of chest trauma. On the one hand, rib and sternum fractures are accurately diagnosable, on the other hand, local hematomas, pleural effusions, and pneumothoraces are also detectable (Mathis 1996; Mathis 1997).

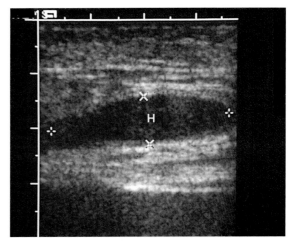

Fig. 2.1. A subcutaneous hematoma (*H*) following blunt trauma. The generally hypoechoic region of the hematoma is composed of thin, hazy internal echoes; echogenic connective tissue surrounding the region

2.1
Soft-Tissue Lesions

Hematomas

As a result of the number of erythrocytes and the grade of organization – usually in connection with the age of the lesion – hematomas can present with varying echo patterns (Fig. 2.1). Sometimes, fine, hazy, central echoes are found, while in rare cases transitional forms to denser echoes can appear. Organized hematomas can look very inhomogeneous.

Abscesses

Cell count and composition of the abscess can result in different central structures. Central parts of abscesses can look similar to hematomas; a differentiation is sometimes difficult because transitional forms, such as infected hematomas, can appear. An important diagnostic criteria is the presence or absence of a capsular formation in different stages, which is highly suggestive of abscesses, while central structures often display movement (Fig. 2.2).

Lipomas

The echogenicity of lipomas depends on cellular fat content and impedance differences in the interstitial tissue. The sonographic texture can vary from echo-poor to relatively echo-rich forms. The borderline to the surrounding tissue can be incomplete (Figs. 2.3a, 2.4).

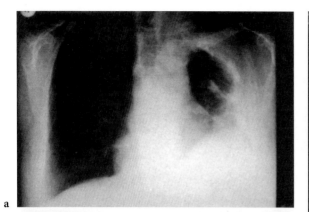

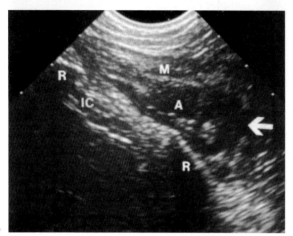

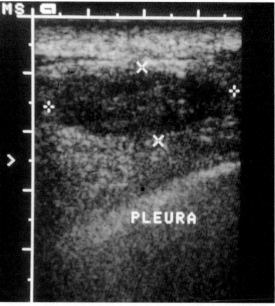

Fig. 2.3. Subcutaneous lipoma, here hypoechoic and sharply delineated. The echogenicity of lipomas depends ultimately on the fat content of cells and the intervening connective tissue. Lipomas may be of different echogenicity

Fig. 2.2. a The chest radiograph of this woman with recurrent bouts of fever only reveals old, scarred post-tuberculotic changes. b The ultrasound image shows a "cold" tuberculotic abscess (A) measuring 30 × 20 mm in size, between the pectoral muscle (M) and rib (R), or intercostal space (IC). The diagnosis was first made by sonography – targeted fine-needle puncture – which showed evidence of acid-proof rod bacteria, and was subsequently confirmed at surgery

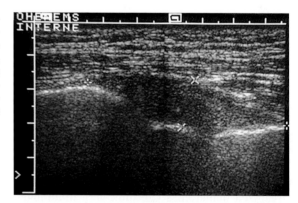

Fig. 2.4. Fibrolipoma in the parietal pleura. The patient was referred because of a suspected peripheral lung carcinoma. On sonography, the tumor could be allocated to the chest wall, based on the gliding pleura. The diagnosis was confirmed by ultrasound-guided biopsy. The tumor had remained constant in size over a 6-year period

Malignancies (Sarcomas, Metastases)

The main criterion in the detection of a malignancy is the characterization of an infiltrative growth pattern. Echo-poor textures can be combined with inhomogeneous echo-rich patterns. Color Doppler sonography can often be very useful in the differential diagnosis of echo-poor lesions suspected of being malignant. The type of vascularizations and morphology of the vessel formation can add important information (Fig. 2.5). In the case of US-guided punctures, it is important to have a good knowledge of the grades of vascularization. Localization in close proximity to the US transducer is optimal for obtaining histologically conclusive tissue probes.

2.2 Lymph Nodes (Inflammatory Lymph Nodes, Lymph Node Metastases)

Lymph nodes can be verified in almost all palpable structures. There are some papers dealing with the problem of predicting the dignity of lesions in relation to sonomorphology (Bruneton et al. 1986; Hergan et al. 1994, 1996). The diagnostic possibilities are rapidly increasing with the improved resolution of B-mode imaging and, of course, with better Doppler techniques and the use of signal enhancing agents (Chang et al. 1994; Table 2.1).

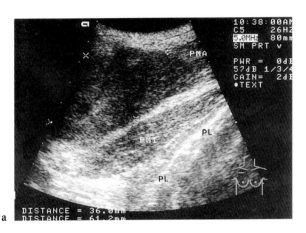
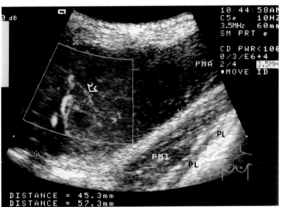

Fig. 2.5a, b. Lymphoma of the muscle in a 20-year-old patient who experienced pain in the chest wall during bodybuilding. Clinically, the patient had a hardening and swelling in the region of the pectoral muscle on the right side. **a** On sonography, a hypoechoic transformation of lateral portions of the pectoralis major, which was interpreted as hemorrhage on the B-mode image. **b** Evidence of marked vascularization of the lesion on color Doppler sonography, with atypical vessels (corkscrew, variations in caliber, high-velocity signals). The surgical biopsy revealed a non-Hodgkin's lymphoma of the pectoral musculature

Table 2.1. Sonomorphology of lymph nodes

	Inflammatory	Malignant lymphoma	Lymph node metastases
Form	Oval/elongated	Round, oval	Round
Margin	Smooth	Smooth	Irregular
Demarcation	Sharp	Sharp	Blurred
Growth	Moniliform (bead-like)	Expansive	Infiltrative
Mobility	Good	Good, moderate	Poor
Echogenicity	Hypoechoic margin "Signs of hilar fat"	Hypoechoic, cystic	Inhomogeneous echoes
Vascularization	Regular, central	Irregular	Corkscrew-like

Establishing the dignity lesions on the basis of sonomorphological criteria should be done so very carefully and must not be overestimated. A definitive diagnosis can only be made on the basis of a histological examination following puncture or on the basis of disease course. In clinical practice, changes in sonomorphological patterns are of extreme interest. Whether in malignant disease or inflammatory processes, therapeutic success can be achieved by means of US follow-up.

Inflammatory Lymph Nodes

Inflammatory lymph nodes seldom exceed 20 mm in size. Usually, they are clearly demarcated and triangular or oblong in shape (Fig. 2.6). In the case of lymphadenitis, a pearl necklace-like formation along the anatomical lymph node stations is very typical. According to the anatomical form, there is often an echo-rich central zone called the "hilar fat sign" and corresponds to the fatty and connecting tissue in the central region of the lymph node. This sign is particularly visible during the healing phase of inflammatory processes (Fig. 2.7). The area showing a sharp demarcation from the surround-

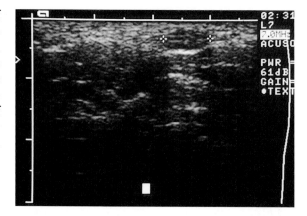

Fig. 2.7. Healing lymph node in mononucleosis. The margin is still hypoechoic, in the center the "hilar fat sign"

ing tissue is echo-poor. Vessels are detectable in this echo-poor area by means of color Doppler sonography. The lymph node hilus with arterial and venous vessels is also often seen.

Lymph Node Metastases

Lymph node metastases mostly look inhomogeneous; often echo-rich parts dominate. The borders to the surrounding tissue is not sharp, an aggressive growth pattern is characterized by infiltration

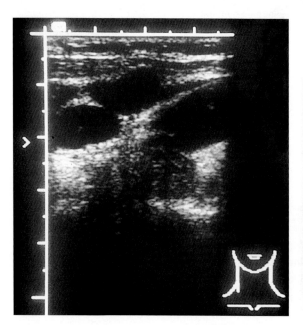

Fig. 2.6. Inflammatory lymph nodes arranged in a chain-of-pearls fashion; hypoechoic in the acute phase

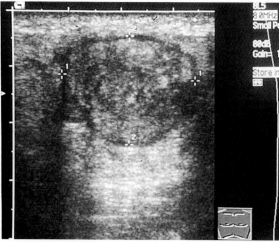

Fig. 2.8. Lymph node metastasis of an epidermoid lung carcinoma. Invasive growth into the surroundings. On palpation, there was markedly reduced mobility. The affected lymph node itself is marked by inhomogeneous echoes

of muscles and vessels (Fig. 2.8; Gritzmann et al. 1990). The size of lymph nodes is not a particularly good criterion for differentiation, but metastases can exceed the maximal inflammatory lymph node diameter of 20 mm. Important is the round shape that is typical for metastases. Lymph node metastases are very good parameters to assess the effectiveness of therapy. Lymph nodes can persist even during the course of chemo- or radiotherapy.

Reactive inflammatory lymph nodes are occasionally also found in the surrounding area of metastases sometimes. Nonpalpable lymph nodes are detectable by ultrasound, particularly in the axilla. US is extremely important in particular at the preoperative stage for the staging process, and also during follow-up examinations of breast cancer, and should be recommended generally (Bruneton et al. 1984; Hergan et al. 1996; Figs. 2.9 a, b, 2.10).

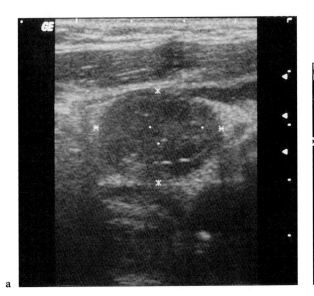

a

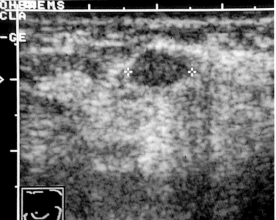

Fig. 2.10. Nonpalpable axillary lymph node metastasis 7 mm in size, in the presence of breast carcinoma

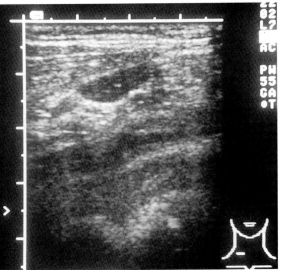

b

Fig. 2.9. **a** Cervical lymph node metastasis of a large-cell lung carcinoma. **b** After two cycles of chemotherapy, this lymph node metastasis has resolved. The present image is that of a reactive lymph node

Malignant Lymphomas

An homogeneous, echo poor, and sharply demarcated shape is typical for malignant lymphomas. Centrocytic malignant lymphomas or Hodgkin lymphomas can present as almost lacking echoes and cyst-like. Malignant lymphomas are round, oval, but seldom triangular (Figs. 2.11, 2.12). Lymph nodes on both sides of a vessel ("sandwich") is also very typical for malignant lymphomas.

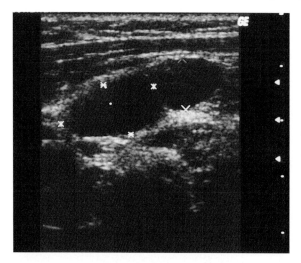

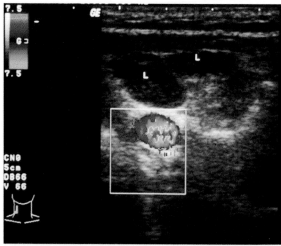

Fig. 2.11. Cervical Hodgkin's lymphoma in stage I. Its resolution under radiotherapy could be followed well by sonography

Fig. 2.12. Centrocytic non-Hodgkin's lymphoma. The oval, homogenous, smoothly margined lymph nodes are seen as anechoic cysts

2.3
Lesions of the Bony Chest

Rib and Sternum Fractures

Radiological chest fracture diagnosis is often difficult, especially in terms of distinguishing a fracture from a contusion. Chest lesions, however, are eminently visible on sonographically (Dubs-Kunz 1992 und 1996, Fenkl et al. 1991, Bitschnau et al. 1997; Table 2.2). One of the advantages of US in chest trauma examination is its ability to detect hematomas, pleural effusions, and lung contusions in addition to the fracture and fracture fragments. In everyday practice, it has proved wise to follow the patient's indications regarding where pain is maximal. In most cases, the diagnosis of a fracture can be established very quickly. Assuming the patient is not dyspneic, the ventral region can be examined with the patient in a supine position, the dorsal region in the upright sitting position. Having the patient place one hand on his/her neck is also useful since this maneuver displaces the scapula laterally, making those parts of the chest wall visible that are normally hidden.

If the fracture is larger than the lateral resolution of the US equipment used, it is sonographically detectable. An indirect fracture sign is the appearance of reverberation artifacts behind the non-dislocated fracture line, known as the "lighthouse

Table 2.2. Sonographic signs of rib and sternum fractures

Direct signs	Indirect signs
At the site of pain	Accompanying hematoma
Cortical gap	"Lighthouse/chimney phenomenon"
Cortical step	Accompanying pleural effusion
	Accompanying pneumothorax
	Accompanying lung contusion foci

or chimney" phenomenon; the artifacts appear on the outer edges of the fracture fragments and reach downwards perpendicularly. The sonomorphological criteria for rib and sternum fractures are more or less the same: a cortical gap or cortical step (Fig. 2.13), indirectly a hematoma, chimney phenomenon, or a pleural effusion (Fig. 2.14).

A sound knowledge of anatomy and possible anatomical variants is important in dealing with sternal fractures. Thus, care should be taken not to misinterpret the normal cortical interruption in the area of the synchondrosis of the manubrium and corpus sterni as a fracture. One should also bear in mind the possibility of various absent bone-process fusions, although these seldom occur.

In follow-up examinations, a local hematoma can be identified initially as an echo-free or echo-poor

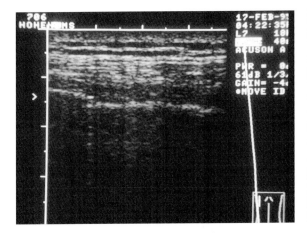

Fig. 2.13. Rib fracture with a step formation (a shift in the uniformity of the rib) of 2 mm. The fracture was not seen on the radiograph

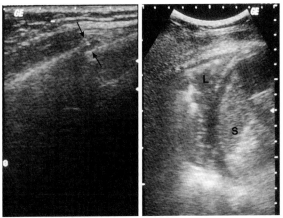

Fig. 2.15. In this multiple rib fracture (*arrows*), one of the fractured ribs is seen on the left side. The right portion of the image reveals an extensive lung contusion focus and a narrow subpulmonary pleural effusion. *L*, liver; *S*, spleen

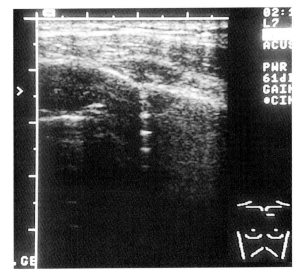

Fig. 2.14. Non-dislocated rib fracture that becomes vaulted on slight pressure. This results in a characteristic "lighthouse" or "chimney" phenomenon. Furthermore, there is a small accompanying hematoma

hem. The subsequent build-up of callus is characterized by organization and concentration. The initial calcification results in fine acoustic shadows, or even complete ossification. Once scar formation is completed, only a hump in the still strong cortical reflex can be seen (Friedrich et al. 1994; Riebel et al. 1995). Abnormal healing processes can be detected in the same way. The first

signs of opacification and ossification occur in weeks 3–4; restitution to the full is usually complete after months.

Some papers attribute great importance to chest sonography in traumatology (Leitgeb et al. 1990; Mariacher-Gehler and Michel 1994). In addition to the information obtained in normal X-ray examinations, chest US can often provide important complementary information (Griffith et al 1999). In a random group of patients with suspected rib fractures, it was found that twice as many fractures could be detected sonographically compared to the number detected with conventional X-ray, including target shots (Bitschnau et al. 1997). Particular advantages were found in the assessment of the ventral region. However, X-ray proved better for the examination of rib fractures combined with clavicular fractures. Of particular importance to the patient is the difference in the period of time they will be unable to return to work depending on whether a rib fracture or a contusion is diagnosed. If there is severe chest trauma, the extent of any accompanying pleural effusion and lung contusion (Fig. 2.15) can easily be quantified and therapeutic modifications can be made immediately. Thus, the use of US in emergency units is of great value (Walz and Muhr 1990; Wischofer et al. 1995).

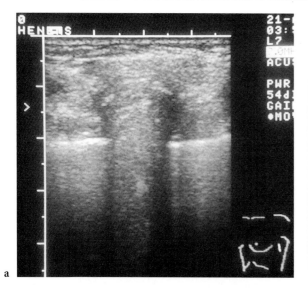

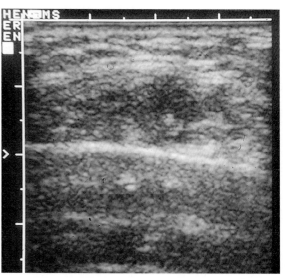

a

b

Fig. 2.16. a Cross-section through an osteolytic rib metastasis in pleuropulmonary adenocarcinoma. **b** Longitudinal section through this metastasis. The rib is distended, the cortical reflex largely destroyed, the echo texture of the metastasis is inhomogeneous. The pathological echo transmission allows the pleura to be visualized

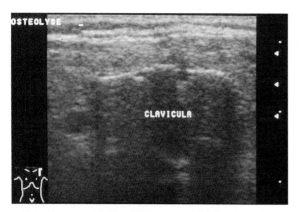

Fig. 2.17. Osteolytic metastasis in the left clavicle. Only the cortical reflex is fragmented here. The extent of the lesion was seen better on the radiograph in this case

Osteolyses

Osteolyses are usually the result of metastases, presenting as a disturbed or destroyed cortical reflex with pathological US transmission (Fig. 2.16 a, 2.17). Osteolyses are usually well-demarcated round or oval lesions. The echo structure is sometimes echo-poor and hazy. Using color Doppler sonography, corkscrew-like vessel neoformations can be found (Fig. 2.18). If a histological diagnosis is necessary, a US-guided puncture is the way of choice. During the course of therapy, size, shape and structure of osteolyses as with plasmocytomas (Fig. 2.19), small cell bronchus carcinomas, as well as prostate or breast cancers can be used as follow-up parameters. The grade of infiltration of the chest wall and the relationship to surrounding subclavian vessels in peripheral bronchus carcinomas is important in Pancoast tumors and sometimes more accurately assessed sonographically than using computed tomography (Fig. 2.20).

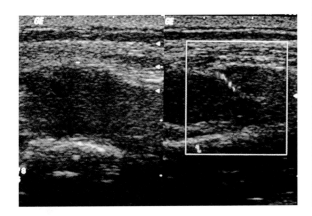

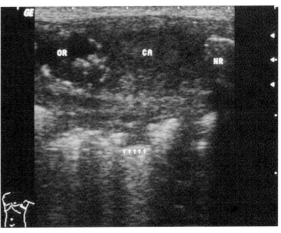

Fig. 2.18. Invasion of a rib by a highly malignant non-Hodgkin's lymphoma with pathological neoformation of vessels on color Doppler sonography. The diagnosis was made by ultrasound-guided puncture

Fig. 2.20. Peripheral lung carcinoma invading the chest wall. *CA*, carcinoma; *OR*, osteolytic rib; *NR*, normal rib. Tumor cones can be seen in the deeper regions (*arrows*)

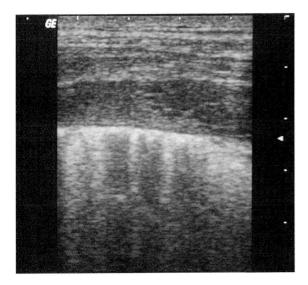

Fig. 2.19. Plasmazytoma. Entirely re-formed rib, with somewhat inhomogeneous echoes and pathological echo transmission up to the pleura

Summary

The detection of lymph nodes and careful interpretation of dignity is one of the main indications for chest wall sonography. In the case of therapeutic consequences, all unclear lesions of the chest wall are well accessible to US-guided puncture for histological diagnosis. The risk of puncture is very low due to the proximity to the US probe. When follow-up examinations are necessary, they can reproduced easily. Both rib and sternum fractures are readily detectable. In addition to the fact that US fracture diagnosis is more sensitive than conventional X-ray, accompanying soft-parts processes, pleural effusions, and hematomas can be also be visualized.

References

Bitschnau R, Gehmacher O, Kopf A, Scheier M, Mathis G (1997) Ultraschalldiagnostik von Rippen- und Sternumfrakturen. Ultraschall Med 18:158–161

Bruneton JN, Caramella E, Hery M, Aubanel D, Manzino JJ, Picard L (1986) Axillary lymph node metastases in breast cancer: Preoperative Detection with US. Radiology 158:325–326

Bruneton JN, Caramella E, Aubanel D, Hery M, Ettore F, Boublil JL, Picard L (1984) Ultrasound versus clinical examination for axillary lymph node involvement in breast cancer. Ultrasound 153:297

Chang DB, Yuan A, Yu CJ, Luh KT, Kuo SH, Yang PC (1994) Differentiation of benign and malinant cervical lymph nodes with color doppler sonography. Am J Roentgenol 162:965–968

Dubs-Kunz B (1992) Sonographische Diagnostik von Rippenfrakturen. In: Anderegg A, Despland P, Henner H, Otto R (Hrsg) Ultraschalldiagnostik '91, Springer, Berlin Heidelberg New York Tokyo, pp 268–273

Dubs-Kunz B (1996) Sonography of the chest wall. Eur J Ultrasound 3:103–111

Fenkl R, v. Garrel T, Knappler H (1992) Diagnostik der Sternumfraktur mit Ultraschall – Eine Vergleichsstudie zwischen Radiologie und Ultraschall. In: Anderegg A, Despland P, Henner H, Otto R: Ultraschalldiagnostik '91, Springer, Berlin Heidelberg New York Tokyo, pp 274–279

Friedrich RE, Volkenstein RJ (1994) Diagnose und Repositionskontrolle von Jochbogenfrakturen. Ultraschall Med 15:213–216

Griffith JF, Rainer TH, Ching AS, Law KL, Cocks RA, Metreweli C (1999) Sonography compared with radiography in revealing acute rib fracture. Am J Roentgenol 173:1603–1609

Gritzmann N, Grasl MC, Helmer M, Steiner E (1990) Invasion of the carotid artery and jugular vein by lymph node metastases: Detection with sonography. Am J Roentgenol 154:411–414

Hergan K, Amann T, Oser W (1994) Sonopathologie der Axilla: Teil II. Ultraschall Med 15:11–19

Hergan K, Haid A, Zimmermann G, Oser W (1996) Preoperative axillary sonography in brest cancer: Value of the method when done routinely. Ultraschall Med 17:14–17

Leitgeb N, Bodenteich A, Schweighofer F, Fellinger M (1990) Sonographische Frakturdiagnostik. Ultraschall Med 11:206–209

Mariacher Gehler S, Michel BA (1994) Sonography: A simple way to visualize rib fractures (letter) Am J Roentgenol 163:1268

Mathis G (1996) Lungen und Pleurasonographie. 2nd ed, Springer, Berlin Heidelberg New York Tokyo, 1996

Mathis G (1997) Thoraxsonography – Part I: Chest wall and pleura. Ultrasound Med Biol 23:1141–1153

Riebel T, Nasir R (1995) Sonographie geburtstraumatischer Extremitätenläsionen. Ultraschall in Med 16:196–199

Sakai F, Sone S, Kiyono K et al. (1990) High resolution ultrasound of the chest wall. Fortschr Röntgenstr 153:390–394

Szuzuki N, Saitoh T Kitamura S (1993) Tumor invasion of the chest wall in lung cancer: diagnosis with US. Radiology 187:39–42

Walz M, Muhr G (1990) Sonographische Diagnostik beim stumpfen Thoraxtrauma. Unfallchirurg 93:359–363

Wischofer E, Fenkl R, Blum R (1995) Sonographischer Nachweis von Rippenfrakturen zur Sicherung der Frakturdiagnostik. Unfallchirurg 98:296–300

3 The Pleura

J. REUSS

Besides the chest wall, the pleura is the thoracic structure which can be reached most easily and best depicted sonographically. With the appropriate examination method, the whole costal and diaphragmatic pleura can be visualized. The visceral pleura, which is hidden behind the ribs, can be shifted to the intercostal space by means of breathing maneuvers. From the jugular direction, the upper, forward mediastinum with its parts of the pleura can be captured. The lower, rear mediastinal and paravertebral sections of the pleura are not usually not discernible on transthoracic sonography. According to estimates based on transverse sections of the thorax using computed tomography, at least 60%–70% of the pleura surface can be visualized sonographically (Reuss 1996). Most diseases of the pleura affect the costal and diaphragmatic pleural segments. The value of color duplex sonography of the pleura, however, has not been systematically evaluated, but it is helpful in differentiating tumor-like lesions and infiltrations, especially in the thoracic wall and in the lung.

3.1
Normal Pleura

The normal pleura is only 0.2–0.4 mm thick and hence at the resolution limits of even modern ultrasound systems (Bittner et al. 1995). Due to the different acoustic impedance at the interface of the pleural sheets, a depiction is nonetheless sonographically feasible. The parietal pleura shows as a fine echogenic line, the pleural cavity as an echo-free to highly hypoechogenic parallel band (Börner et al. 1987). The actual thickness of the pleural sheets is exaggerated in that process.

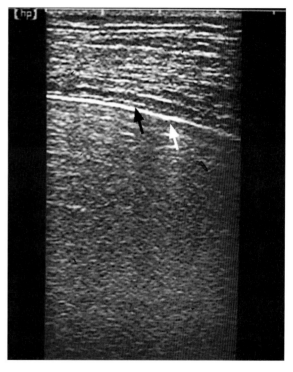

Fig. 3.1. Chest wall with normal smooth pleura. The apparently thicker visceral pleura (*white arrow*) is an artifact caused by the total reflection at the air-filled lung. Small comet-tail-artifacts. Between the pleural sheets one can identify the echo-free pleural space (*black arrow*). The hypoechogenic extrapleural fatty layer between parietal pleura and chest wall

The essentially finer visceral pleura is submerged in the thick line of total reflection of the ultrasound at the air-filled lung (Fig. 3.1). As soon as the peripheral lung – due to a pathological process – is free of air, the actual visceral pleura can be marked-off as a fine echogenic line (Fig. 3.2). In day-to-day ultrasound practice, the described line

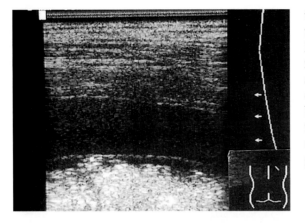

Fig. 3.2. Subpleural infiltrations in a patient with pulmonary embolism and pleural effusion. These infiltrations make the visceral pleura distinguishable from the total reflection band at the air-filled parts of the lung. Visceral and parietal pleura of the same thickness and equal echogenicity

of total reflection is know as the visceral pleura. The fine hypoechogenic band outside the parietal pleura seems to correspond to the extrapleural fatty layer (Bittner et al. 1995).

Comet tail artifacts also form on normal pleura (Fig. 3.1). The respiratory shift of the lung against the parietal pleura can be observed easily, even without comet tail artifacts. The respiratory movement of the lung is greatest dorsolateral and caudal. Patients suffering from asthma or emphysema display, even under normal conditions, minimal respiratory lung movement only. The absence of respiratory shift is a diagnostic sign of inflammatory or tumorous adhesions of the pleura. Due to interposed air, no respiratory shift in the case of pneumothorax can be seen. Sonography, being a real-time application, again has a major advantage over other imaging modalities.

3.2
Pleural Effusion

Although pleural effusions could be observed very early on with B-image sonography, chest radiography is still the main method of choice for establishing the presence of or following up pleural effusions (Joyner et al. 1967). Sonography, however, is more suitable for proving or excluding the existence of pleural effusions, as well as for estimating their volume.

Pleural effusions are echo-free since they are liquid formations. The pleura sharply delineates the effusions (Fig. 3.3). Large effusions can be verified easily by ultrasound, whereas smaller effusions between the chest wall and diaphragm or parallel to the pleura in the delimitation to the hypoechogenic swelling of the pleura are hard to distinguish (Figs. 3.4, 3.5).

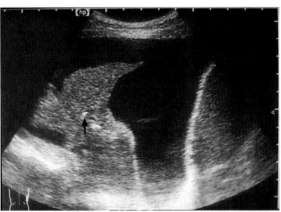

Fig. 3.3. Large, almost echo-free pleural effusion. The echoes in the depth are artifacts. Compressed lung with only a small volume of residual air in the central bronchi (*arrow*)

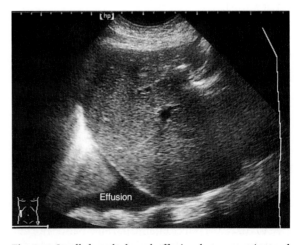

Fig. 3.4. Small dorsal pleural effusion between spine and diaphragm in a transhepatic view

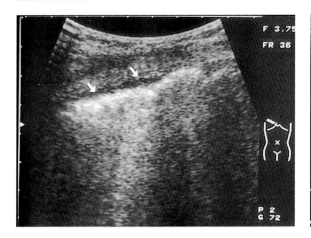

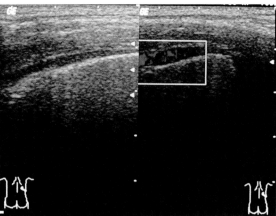

Fig. 3.5. Very small, narrow pleural effusion (*arrows*). The changing shape of the effusion area during the examination is not consistent with a circumscribed pleural thickening

Fig. 3.6. Small effusion in the costophrenic angle. The color Doppler signals in the effusion originate from the pulse- and respiration-synchronous shifting of the fluid and characterize the not completely echo-free formation as an effusion

The effusion is echo-free, displays a change of form during breathing and sometimes septa or floating echoes occur. Additionally, a color Doppler signal can be caused by the shifting of liquid in the effusion synchronous with respiration (Fig. 3.6). One study showed that 10% of false positive results could be corrected and the specificity of sonographic verification of small effusions rose from 68% to 100% due to the use of this color Doppler signal in addition to the B-mode examination (Wu et al. 1994). There are no false positive results for medium or large effusions, since atelectases, a raised diaphragm, tumors, or pleural fibrosis are sonographically unmistakable, whereas they are unclearly delineated on X-ray. The sonographic exclusion of pleural effusions is possible, with the exception of effusions captured in the interlobar space (Fig. 3.7).

On average, a minimum of 150 ml of pleural effusion is required to enable detection on standard X-ray with the patient in a standing position (Collins et al. 1972). In contrast, effusions of as little as 5 ml can be identified without problem sonographically laterodorsal in the angle between the chest wall and the diaphragm with patients in either a standing or sitting position (Gryminski et al. 1976). Sonography is far more reliable at verifying pleural effusions (sensitivity 100%; specificity 99.7%) than conventional X-ray of the thorax with the patient in a standing position (sensitivity 71%; specificity 98.5%) (Goecke and Schwerk 1990).

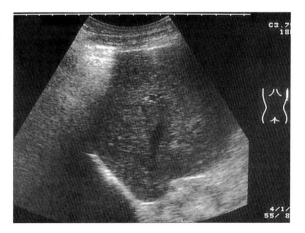

Fig. 3.7. No fluid between liver and lung, thus excluding a free-floating effusion. To exclude an effusion in the pleura altogether, the entire pleura must be examined

By turning the supine patient slightly sidewards, small dorsal effusions can also be identified. The examination can be carried out at the bedside and repeated anytime for follow-up purposes. Using X-ray, effusions can be verified in only half the number of patients in a supine position. Even large effusions on both sides and leaking dorsally cannot be recognized (Table 3.1). Effusion and atelectasis cannot be distinguished from one another radiologically, often leading to an overestimation of the volume of effusion shown on X-ray (Kelbel et al. 1990).

Table 3.1. Evidence of pleural effusions on chest X-ray in supine patients. Of 110 single examinations on 50 patients, effusions were correctly identified sonographically in every case. (From Kelbel et al. 1990)

Pleural effusion	Right	Left	Both sides
Correct evidence	Sensitivity 47% Specificity 71%	Sensitivity 55% Specificity 93%	Sensitivity 38%
Correct volumes	57%	24%	
Volume <200 ml	Sensitivity 23%	Sensitivity 30%	
Volume >500 ml	Sensitivity 83%	Sensitivity 73%	
Additional atelectases	Sensitivity 7%	Sensitivity 13.5	

Table 3.2. Formulae to estimate the volume of pleural effusions

Formula	Publication
LSF (cm²) × U (cm) × 0.89 = E (ml)	Lorenz et al. 1988
QSF (cm²) × H (cm) × 0.66 = E (ml)	Kelbel et al. 1990
LH (cm) × 90 = E (ml), correlation coefficient $r = 0.68$	Goecke und Schwerk 1990
LH (cm) + SH (cm) × 70 = E (ml), correlation coefficient $r = 0.87$	Goecke und Schwerk 1990
D (mm) × 47.6–837 = E (ml)	Eibenberger et al. 1994

D, thickness of effusion layer, supine position; *E*, effusion volume empirical factors; *H*, effusion height; *LH*, lateral height of effusion, sitting position; *LSF*, median of planes of longitudinal sections through the effusion in six positions; *QSF*, horizontal plane through the effusion; *SH*, median subpulmonary height of effusion, sitting position; *U*, circumference of the hemithorax.

Sonographic methods to estimate the volume of pleural effusion differ in terms of their accuracy and practicability. For practical purposes, the method published by Goecke and Schwerk (1990) is easy to perform and saves time (Table 3.2).

An estimated result differing by less than 10% of the actual volume can be achieved by multiplying the median planes of longitudinal sections in six positions from parasternal to paravertebral with the determined circumference of the hemithorax and the empirical factor of 0.89 (Lorenz et al. 1988).

Another method, which achieves a good correlation of measured data and actual volume of the effusion, is to multiply the cross plane, determined planimetrically, with the maximum height of the effusion and the empirical factor 0.66 (Kelbel et al. 1990) (Figs. 3.8, 3.9).

In addition, the volume of a pleural effusion has been estimated using multiple empirical formulas including the lateral height of the effusion, the sub-pulmonary height of the effusion, or the thickness of the mantle of the effusion around the lungs.

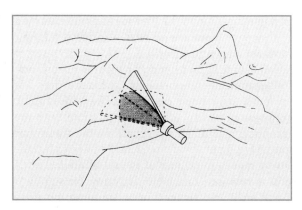

Fig. 3.8. An estimation of the volume of pleural effusions in the supine patient. (From Börner et al. 1987)

An easy to perform method which is also adequate for general purposes measures the lateral height of the effusion at the chest wall. The determined value in centimeters, multiplied by the empirical factor 90 amounts to the effusion volume in milli-

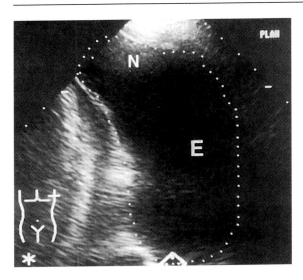

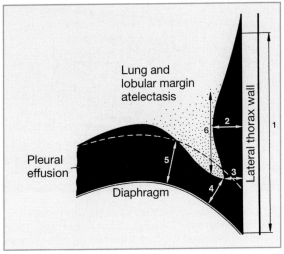

Fig. 3.9. An example of effusion planimetry. The cardiac effusion in a supine, intensive-care patient can be well estimated, followed up and documented. *E*, effusion; *N*, noise artifacts

Fig. 3.10. Pleural effusion volumetry in sitting patients. Useful parameters include the maximal extent of effusion (*1*), the basal distance between lung and diaphragm (*4*), and the subpulmonary effusion height (*5*). The thickness of the lateral mantle of the effusion (*2*), the distance between the basal lung atelectasis and the chest wall (*3*), and the height of the basal atelectasis (*6*) are not suitable parameters for estimation of the volume of effusion. (From Goecke and Schwerk 1990)

liters ($r = 0.68$). Small effusions will be overestimated using this approximation formula. The total of the basal lung–diaphragm distance and the lateral height of the effusion multiplied by 70 will result in more precise estimates ($r = 0.87$) (Figs. 3.10, 3.11) Goecke and Schwerk 1990).

The estimation of the volume of a pleural effusion based on sonography is more precise than the estimation based on radiology. In a study, the radiological volume estimation – compared to the sonographic one – was correct in 57% of cases concerning the right hemithorax and correct in only 24% of cases concerning the left hemithorax (Kelbel et al. 1990). The sonographic volume estimation correlates closer with the actual punctured volume than the radiological method ($r = 0.80$ vs. $r = 0.58$, $p < 0.05$; Eibenberger et al. 1994).

In the supine patient, the sonographic measurement of the thickness of the dorsal fluid layer is closer to the actual volume, determined by thoracocenteses, than the estimated volume, based on radiologic examination. A simplified approximation is $y = 50\ x - 800$, where y represents the sought volume of the effusion and x the thickness of the effusion in millimeters measured at a right angle to the chest wall (original formula $y = 47.6\ x - 837$; Eibenberger et al. 1994). The deviation of the estimated results from the actual volume of the effusion can be considerable.

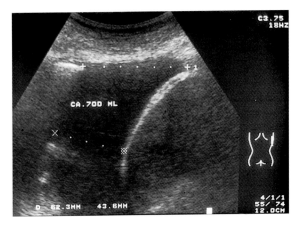

Fig. 3.11. A simple estimation of effusion volume by measuring the height of the subpulmonary effusion and the maximum height. Estimated volume 700 ml, actual volume 800 ml. (From Goecke and Schwerk 1990)

The type of pleural effusion is also important for diagnostic purposes. Transudates contain no components which could serve as ultrasound reflectors and are therefore echo-free. Exudates, with their

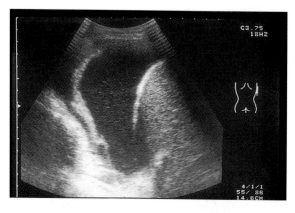

Fig. 3.12. Echogenic protein-rich effusion in a patient with an IgA plasmocytoma. In contrast to artificial echoes, these echoes are swirling pulse- and respiration-synchronous in the effusion during real-time-examination

high protein content and cell-containing or sanguineous effusions often appear echogenically in ultrasound images (Fig. 3.12). Under real-time conditions, echoes float or swirl with respiration and heartbeat, making circular movements, and can hence be distinguished easily from the echoes of artifacts.

According to prospective studies, transudates are always echo-free, whereas exudates can be both echo-free and echogenic. Empyemas or hemothoraces display relatively homogeneous echogenicity. Additional findings such as septation or nodular pleural changes always indicate an exudate (Yang et al. 1992). Very rarely, transudates can be faintly echogenic. There is no explanation for this ultrasound phenomenon (Reuss 1996). Hence, if there is diagnostic interest, the pleural effusion should always be punctured. US-guided percutaneous transthoracic needle aspiration biopsy and, if necessary, even thoracocentesis, can be performed on critically ill patients at their bedside (Yu et al. 1992).

The effusion fluid should then be examined using chemical, bacteriological, cytological, and, if necessary, virological or immunological methods. Very often, additional information relating to the primary disease can be obtained on the basis of these methods (Sahn 1988).

3.3
Solid Pleural Changes

The only visible reactions of the pleura to disease are exudation of fluid and edema. Pleural edema can appear diffuse, circumscribed, band-like, nodular, regular, irregular, hypoechogenic, or complexly structured. If the lung is still shifting with respiration, the swelling can unambiguously be associated with the parietal or visceral pleura, depending on whether the lung is still moving or not.

If the pleural sheets are adhered, the position of the former pleural cavity can often only be guessed at by means of a faintly echogenic, partly interrupted line. Swellings of the pleura occur if something is inflamed or if a primary or secondary tumorous disease exists. From the sonographic structure and form of the pleural swelling, it is not possible to establish its etiology with certainty, even though images such as hypoechogenic nodules are typical signs for metastases (Yang et al. 1992).

Pleuritis

Clinically, pleuritis is difficult to diagnose and often the diagnosis can only be reached by excluding other diseases which cause thoracic pain. Angina pectoris, myocardial infarction, and pain in the bones or nerves are usually the things that spring to mind first. Chest X-rays often show a blurred or even absent contour of the diaphragm. They can also demonstrate an effusion in the pleural recesses, but on the whole these are nonspecific or completely inconspicuous (Loddenkemper 1994).

Most patients with pleuritis have sonographically conspicuous findings of the pleura (Table 3.3).

The parietal pleura is generally hypoechogenically thickened, especially during the early stages of pleuritis (Fig. 3.13) (Bittner et al. 1995). Thickening

Table 3.3. Sonographic findings in pleurisy (frequency). (From Gehmacher et al. 1997)

- Rough appearance and interruption of the normally smooth pleura (89.4%)
- Small subpleural consolidations of between 0.2 and 2.0 cm (63.8%)
- Localized parietal and basal pleural effusions (63.8%)

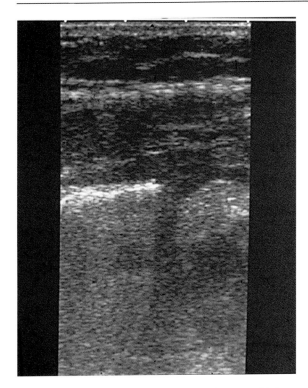

Fig. 3.13. Newly acquired pleurisy with echo-poor thickening of the pleura with nodules, seen in the algetic area of the chest wall

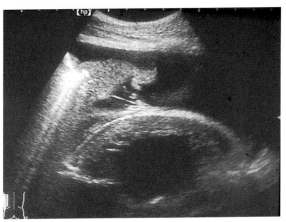

Fig. 3.15. Lung atelectasis, fixed to the pleura near the pericardium by fibrinous bands, inflammatory effusion

of the visceral pleura often involves the surface of the lung tissue, which displays small, round to wedge-shaped areas. Besides the actual swellings of the pleura, fibrinous bands as superimposed layers begin to appear in due course. These fibrinous bands can even be echogenic. They occur in the accompanying effusion as uneven or pronged dips, threads or bands, which – at a later stage of the pleuritis – divide the effusion into numerous cavities by a network of septa (Figs. 3.14–3.16).

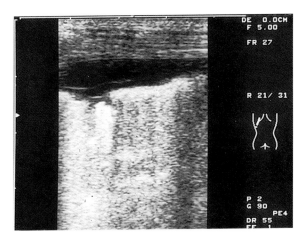

Fig. 3.14. Tuberculous pleurisy without thickening of the parietal pleura, irregular visceral pleura with tiny circumscribed nodules, subpleural pulmonary infiltrations, and fibrinous threads in the effusion. Mycobacterium tuberculosis were found in the effusion

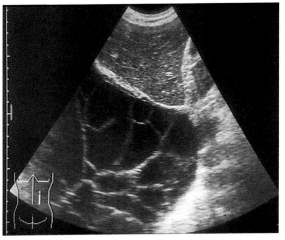

Fig. 3.16. Honeycomb-like appearance of a postinflammatory effusion. In such cases, ultrasound avoids frustrating attempts to perform thoracocentesis with the potential risk of injury

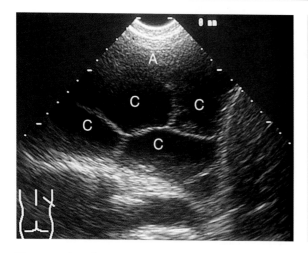

Fig. 3.17. Pleural empyema with several cavities (*C*). The aspirate from different cavities was sometimes purulent, sometimes serous. *A*, artefact

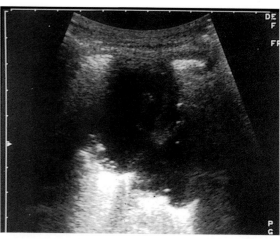

Fig. 3.18. Single cavity of a pleural empyema with a smooth, thin wall. During dynamic examination, the lung showed – as expected – no shift in the area of the empyema

Bacterial pleuritis or, in the later course, bacterial colonization of the septate pleural effusion, e. g., by means of an accompanying pneumonia, can cause empyemas to develop, which sometimes develop in only some of the cavities. Any attempt to puncture septate pleural effusions for therapeutic purposes, i. e., to relieve the patient from breathing difficulties, is usually unsuccessful. Prior sonographic examination can help to determine a suitable place for diagnostic and therapeutic puncture. The septation of inflammatory effusions is depicted far better using sonography than computed tomography.

Color Doppler sonography of the expected hyperemia in pleurisy has, so far, proved to be rather disappointing (Fig. 3.17). Intensified vascularization could be observed in only 23.4% of cases and hence this method is limited in its application as a diagnostic signal (Gehmacher et al. 1997).

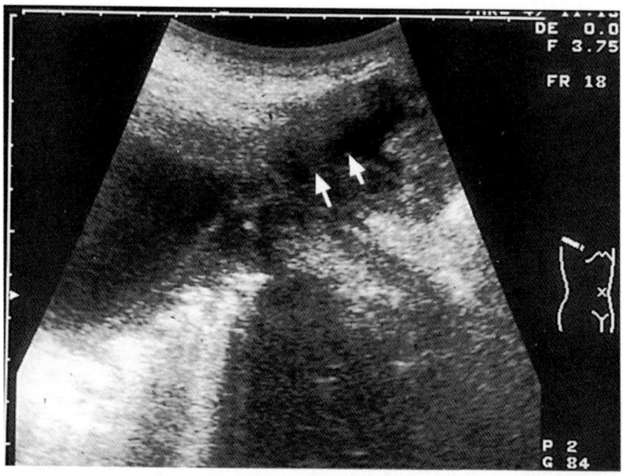

Pleural Empyema

Pleural empyema often look encapsulated, not free floating, and are often faintly to moderately echogenic, relatively homogeneous effusions, whereby the pleura is mostly thickened in a capsule-like fashion (Fig. 3.18). On the computer tomographic images, pleural empyemas have a thinner, more regular, smooth cavity wall compared to peripheral subpleural pulmonary abscess-

Fig. 3.19. Pleural empyema with a thick, but nevertheless smooth wall and clearly visible split pleura. The empyema drained spontaneously by a fistula through the chest wall, surrounded by extensive inflammatory infiltrations (*arrows*)

es (Baber et al. 1980; Layer et al. 1999). The splitting of the pleural sheets around the empyema can also be seen on sonographic images (Figs. 3.19, 3.20). The fibrinous bands and septa, which are easy to detect sonographically, are difficult to delineate on computed tomography. Empyemas mostly display moderately distinctive infiltrations in the adjacent lung, whereas pulmonary abscesses show extended inflammatory infiltrations of the surrounding areas

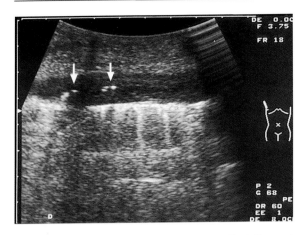

Fig. 3.20. Clearly visible regular and well delineated thickening of the parietal and visceral pleura in an already drained empyema. Small air bubbles in the completely emptied cavity (*arrows*)

and a rather thick wall. Additionally, atelectatic areas of the lung in the surroundings of the pulmonary abscess, which are sonolucent after resorption of the trapped air, add to the impression of a thick, irregularly shaped wall of the pulmonary abscess. Air-filled abscess cavities display a change in air–fluid level as the patient changes his position. This is an almost certain sign of a connection between the cavity and the bronchi, and therefore of an abscess. After attempts to puncture, empyemas can be artificially filled with air. Gas producing bacteria are relatively rare in pleural empyemas.

The radiological signs – obtuse or acute angles between effusion or empyema and chest wall – have proved to be diagnostically insufficient to mark out pulmonary abscesses or adhered pleural effusions, even though these signs can also be found on sonographic images (Fig. 3.18) (Baber et al. 1980; Stark et al. 1983). The sonographically guided puncture provides clarity about the contents of a cavity. In individual cases, a differentiation between pulmonary abscess and pleural empyema can be very difficult. Crucial for the therapy is that one does not drain through ventilated lung and that pleural shifting at the prospective site of the drainage is blocked. Through an adhered pleura, abscesses can be drained without the risk of causing a consecutive empyema.

Benign Pleural Tumors

Benign pleural tumors such as lipomas, schwannomas, chondromas, or benign pleural mesotheliomas are very rare and usually attract attention on chest X-ray as they are mostly unclear, sharply delineated pleural lesions (Theros and Feigin 1977). They account for less than 5% of all pleural tumors (Saito et al. 1988). However, benign pleural tumors are often the reason for further diagnostic measures aimed at excluding pleural metastases or peripheral bronchogenic carcinomas. Benign pleural tumors are moderately echogenic and delineated sharply by a fine capsule. They can displace adjacent structures, but they do not display invasive, destructive growth into their surroundings (Fig. 3.21). It is not always possible to distinguish between displacement and invasion sonographically. Transpleural tumor growth with no respiratory movement of the lung is an indication of malignant growth and infiltration. Small accompanying pleural effusions around the tumor or in the angle between the chest wall and diaphragm can also occur with benign tumors. Sonographic classification of the individual benign pleural tumors is not possible. Histologic classification of benign tumors, based on small fine needle biopsy specimens, or even only on a cytological specimen, is more difficult for the pathologist than to find evidence of a malignancy. Hyperechoic shadowy calcifications point to a benign process. Sonographic density measurements of the tissue as in computer tomography, e.g., to identify fat in lipomas, are not currently available, but they are being developed.

Pleural Metastases

The development of pleural metastases usually parallels that of a pleural effusion. This "sonographic window" makes the detection and depiction of metastases easier. Most metastases are found at the costal pleura or on the diaphragm, as well as in the angle between the diaphragm and the chest wall, i.e., in transthoracically accessible areas – even without an accompanying effusion (Figs. 3.22–3.24).

Pleural metastases are mainly hypoechogenic to moderately echogenic. They are located mainly on the pleura and look like nodular, round-shaped to hemispherical or broad-based polypoid forma-

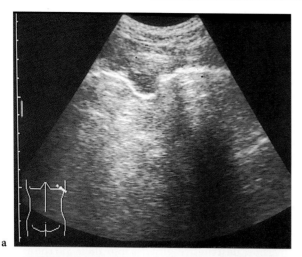

a

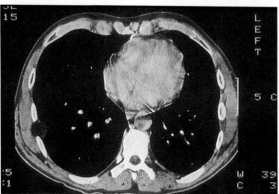

b

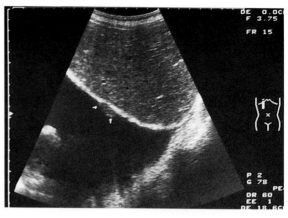

Fig. 3.22. Typical moderately echogenic oval pleural metastasis (*arrows*) in a metastatic breast carcinoma. The diaphragm in the area of the metastasis is already slightly thinned by the infiltration

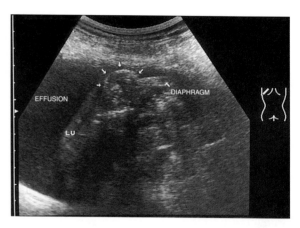

Fig. 3.21. a A small, round, well-delineated tumor in the parietal pleura, the lung shifted along the tumor during respiration. The tumor is isoechogenic with the chest wall musculature. On routine chest-X-ray, an indistinct opacity next to the pleura was discovered. **b** On computed tomography, a well-delineated, fat-isodense tumor was seen, consistent with a pleural lipoma. No biopsy was carried out, but the tumor showed a constant size in follow-up examinations over many years

Fig. 3.23. Hemispheric metastasis, isoechogenic to the diaphragmatic muscle (*arrows*), located on the diaphragmatic pleura, metastatic liposarcoma. Primary localization was in the abdomen. *LU*, lung

Fig. 3.24. Hemispheric hypoechogenic pleural metastasis with poorly delineated lateral processes and chest wall infiltration. Absent pleural effusion. Known breast carcinoma. In such an unusual pleural finding, a peripheral bronchial carcinoma cannot be excluded   ▶

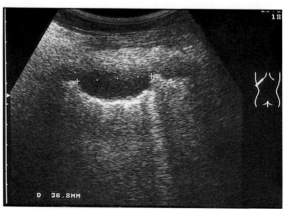

tions, which protrude prominently into the effusion. Depending on the location of the metastases, they can be detected on the screen measuring from 1–2 mm. Large metastases can invade deep into the surrounding tissue, i. e., the lung or chest wall, such that the original point of invasion is no longer visible. Signs of infiltration include a faint, interrupted, or even absent delimitation of the metastasis from its surroundings, or a pseudopodium-like offshoot which, due to its lower echogenicity compared to the chest wall or the diaphragm, is often readily visible (Fig. 3.25). Single, well delineated metastases cannot be distinguished from benign pleural tumors due to their similar sonomorphology. The existence of several similar formations is a very typical finding in pleural metastases and an all but conclusive finding, especially if a corresponding primary disease exists. Hence, confirmation with biopsy may not always be necessary. The transthoracic, sonographically guided needle biopsy contributes essentially to the further diagnosis of a suspected but unknown primary tumor. Pleural metastases are found most frequently with breast cancer or bronchial carcinomas. Single metastases located in the visceral pleura can, sonomorphologically, resemble peripheral bronchial carcinomas (Fig. 3.24). Similar to peripheral bronchial carcinomas, pleural metastases can spread from one pleural sheet to the other and hence lead to concretion of the pleural sheets, accompanied by a lack of respiratory movement of the lung (Suzuki et al. 1993). Extensive or sheet-like infiltrations of the pleura in metastatic carcinomatosis with or without effusion are rarely seen. Sonomorphologically, they are hard to distinguish from the hypoechogenic inflammatory thickening on the one hand, and the tapestry-like mesothelioma on the other. Even needle biopsy can fail to resolve the problem of whether malignant and inflammatory-reactive, fibrinous or sanguineous parts lie next to each other.

Malignant Pleural Mesothelioma

The incidence of asbestos-induced malignant pleural mesothelioma is increasing significantly (Mowé and Tellnes 1995). The period of latency between exposure to asbestos and tumor manifestation can be more than 20 years and hence the number of diseases caused by asbestos is expected to rise within the next 10–20 years even though the use of asbestos has – to a large extent – been disallowed.

Asbestos plaques in the pleura are considered a precursor to mesotheliomas. Asbestos plaques are calcified or noncalcified plateau like thickenings of the pleura which occur mainly in the dorsolateral areas of the parietal pleura. High-risk groups are examined at regular intervals by occupational healthcare specialists. Sonography, with its high local resolution, would be a useful instrument to monitor the pleural changes of these high-risk groups; however, it has not yet been evaluated in major studies. Using preferably high resolution transducers, one can depict the predominantly moderately echogenic swellings of the parietal pleura with its often smooth border and the lung shifting against these plaques during respiration. Not even small effusions should occur together with these plaques. Plaques may also appear as flat formations running out into the normal pleura (Fig. 3.26) (Reuss J, unpublished data).

Mesotheliomas have very irregular, partly angular, unclear borders (Fig. 3.31). In addition to tumor-like formations, mesotheliomas can also present as extensive, tapestry-like growths with nodules (Fig. 3.27).

With a high frequency transducer, the invasion of the chest wall and the diaphragm appears hypo-

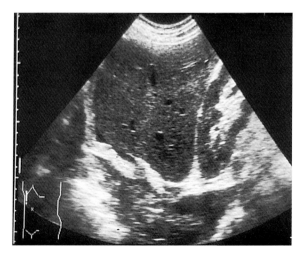

Fig. 3.25. Extended pleural carcinosis in a metastatic bronchial carcinoma with infiltration and penetration of the diaphragm, ascites are already present between the liver and diaphragm. The inhomogeneous structure of the diaphragm and its angular shape are conspicuous signs of malignant infiltration

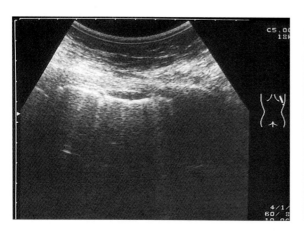

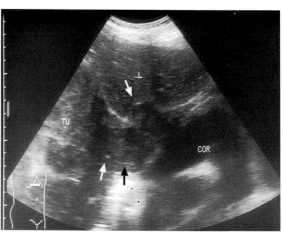

Fig. 3.26. Circumscribed, lenticular, hypoechogenic thickening of the parietal pleura dorsolaterally (pleural plaque), with the lung shifting along the tumor during respiration in a patient with known asbestosis

Fig. 3.28. Advanced pleural mesothelioma with penetration of the diaphragm and infiltration of the cardiac wall. *L*, liver; *TU*, tumor; *COR*, heart

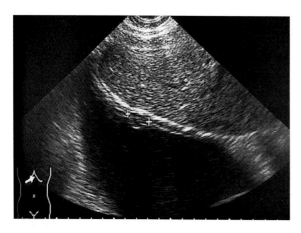

Fig. 3.27. Primary diagnosis of a tapestry-like mesothelioma, spreading over nearly the whole pleura of the right hemithorax with several nodules (between the *crosses*). The patient was referred due to severe dyspnea that developed over 2 days. The chest X-ray showed a white hemithorax. The patient had been exposed to asbestos at work for several decades

echogenic (Fig. 3.28). The invasion soon spreads to the other pleural sheet. The effusions can be echogenic, especially if there is some bleeding.

The diagnosis can be pathohistologically verified during surgery or – preferably – by preoperative biopsy. A biopsy obtained at thoracoscopy is 80%–98% accurate (Börner et al. 1987; Ruffie et al. 1989). In mesotheliomas, the spreading of metasta-

sis along the biopsy channel after sonographically guided biopsy is frequent, especially along the drainage channels after thoracocentesis of large effusions. Nevertheless, it is not always possible to rule out diagnostic and therapeutic punctures and drainages when a mesothelioma can potentially be operated. That said, curative operations of malignant pleural mesotheliomas are out of the question for most of the patients (Sugarbaker et al. 1995).

Computed tomography is the standard method used to diagnose mesotheliomas. Recent preoperative studies have shown that sonographic methods are almost as good as computed tomography or magnetic resonance imaging (Layer et al. 1999). Sonographically detected chest wall infiltrations almost always proved to be true positive, and only a few false positive results occurred.

The region around the diaphragm is, owing to the transverse sections, difficult to examine using computed tomography and can only be judged correctly using reconstruction. As the section angle can be chosen, sonography can help to detect infiltrations and reduce mobility of the diaphragm. Coronary sections of magnetic resonance imaging are not advantageous in this area. Sonographically, the right diaphragm can be accessed a lot better than the left diaphragm. False negative results based on a sonographic examination concern mostly the left half of the diaphragm. The results can be improved if the proximal stomach is filled with water and a consequent examination of the left diaphragm is carried out from ventral, dorsal, and translienal. The sonographic depiction of an invasion of the pericardium is very specific as the sonographic images are moving ones (Fig. 3.28) (Layer et al. 1999).

Transpleural Growth of Tumors

When peripheral lung tumors reach the visceral pleura and cross the pleural space, they infiltrate the parietal pleura and the chest wall. In this difficult situation, any curative surgery will require a chest wall resection. For a surgeon, it is essential to establish the existence of any chest wall infiltration preoperatively. Until now, computed tomography and magnetic resonance imaging were the preferred methods, but it is becoming ever more apparent that a sonographic examination has its advantages. In a retrospective surgically controlled study, sonography (sensitivity 100%, specificity 98%, accuracy 98%) was clearly superior to conventional computed tomography (sensitivity 68%, specificity 66%, accuracy 67%) (Suzuki et al. 1994). A prospective, surgically controlled study comparing ultrasound, computed tomography, and ultrasound guided needle biopsy showed that sonography is superior in the preoperative identification of infiltrations of the chest wall (sensitivity US 76.9%, CT 69.2%, biopsy 61.5%), while its specificity is lower (US 68.8%, CT 75.0%) (Nakano et al. 1994).

Pleural Fibrosis

Large calcified old pleural peels do not usually need any examination other than standard X-ray examination for diagnosis. Noncalcified thickenings manifest themselves radiologically as streaky opacities adjacent to the chest wall or in the angle between chest wall and diaphragm. Sonographically, one can distinguish between solid and liquid formations. A newly developed fibrosis can be so hypoechogenic that – especially if the signal gain is not adjusted optimally – the thickening appears to be echo-free and hence is often misinterpreted as an effusion. Pleural peels with adhered pleural sheets do not show respiratory movement of the lung, which an effusion would still show. The "color-Doppler sign" of narrow effusions of the mantle has already been described (see above).

Even an old fibrosis of many decades standing can be very hypoechogenic, even though fibroses tend to increase their echogenicity with increasing age. Calcifications are shadowy deposits in the pleural fibrosis. Differentiating between calcification and the adjacent air-filled lung is difficult; absent reverberations, however, are an indication of calcification. There are no reliable sonomorphologic criteria to differentiate pleural fibrosis, pleural carcinoma, and mesothelioma (Fig. 3.29). With a color Doppler, cyst-like inclusions, which sometimes exist within the thickening, can be distinguished from thick vessels within the thickening.

Pneumothorax

Reverberation artifacts behind air in the pleura are a lot coarser and more regular than those at the outer surface of the lung (Fig. 3.30). A major criterion of pneumothorax, however, is absent respiratory movement of the lung, which can usually be well observed during a dynamic examination. Asthmatics and patients with distinct emphysema, however, can have low lung shift during respiration even under normal conditions. On ultrasound, no conclusions can be reached regarding thickness of the layer of air or regarding the remaining lung volume. The exclusion of a pneumothorax, e.g., following puncture, can be made sonographically with adequate certainty. A pneumothorax, resulting from a puncture can be detected during the examination as puncture targets behind the parietal pleura are no longer visible once the interposed pleural space is filled with air.

Thorax Trauma

Following thorax injury, a pleural effusion is the symptom which can be best identified sonographically. Fresh, sanguineous effusions are often not, or not yet, echogenic (Fig. 3.31). Exact documentation of the volume of the effusion is important for later follow-up. Other injuries of the chest wall and contusions of the lung are discussed in corresponding chapters of this book. After a thorax trauma, one should always check the pericardium to exclude a traumatic pericardial effusion as a matter of routine.

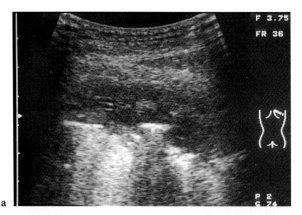

a

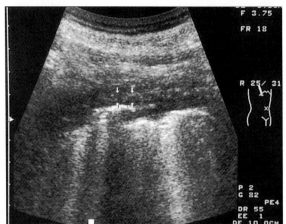

b

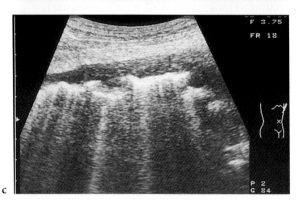

c

Fig. 3.29 a–c. Extended moderate echogenic masses in the pleura with irregularly angular contours are ambiguous and need histological confirmation by biopsy, if other reliable clinical data are not available. a Extended pleural fibrosis in a young woman after multiple operations. A primary pleural peel was erroneously thought to be a tumor and led to the first operation. The growth of the fibrosis afterwards was mistaken for tumor growth. b A slow-growing, radiologically visible noncalcified pleural fibrosis. Due to the clinical suspicion of an occult carcinoma, the patient underwent multiple transthoracic biopsy, each time with only connective and scar tissue. The fibrosis proved later to indeed be the pleural carcinoma of an adenocarcinoma of indistinct primary localization. The area between the *arrows* is believed to be the former pleural fissure line. c An image almost identical to those in (a) an (b), but a histologically proven pleural mesothelioma in an asbestos worker

◄

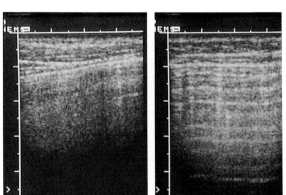

a
b

Fig. 3.30 a, b. Pneumothorax. The left healthy side (a) shows a respiratory shifting pleural reflex and clearly less reverberations. On the side of the pneumothorax (b), the reverberations are intensified and no respiratory shift is visible

►

Fig. 3.31. An emergency examination in the surgical emergency unit performed on a roofer after falling from a roof. The patient had dyspnea and severe thoracic pain on the right side in the area of a visible and palpable fluctuating hematoma. Echo-free, but sanguineous pleural effusion (*PE*) and lung atelectasis. Partly ruptured chest wall with deposition of fluid in the chest wall which fluctuated during dynamic examination, corresponding to the visible and palpable hematoma (*H*)

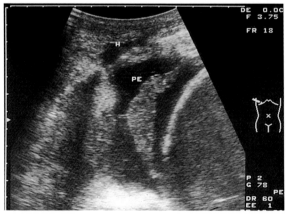

3.4
The Diaphragm

Specific sonographic-scientific publications concerning the diaphragm are rare to date, even though the diaphragm is depicted automatically during abdominal or thoracic sonography, and hence can be assessed both morphologically and functionally.

Anatomically, the diaphragm is symmetric and consists of a pars membranacea which lies more in the dome, as well as of muscular parts which are located towards the ribs, spinal column, and sternum. From these muscular parts, the dorsally inserting diaphragmatic crura next to the lumbar spine can be distinguished. Between these crura run the aorta and the inferior vena cava. Sonographically, the pars membranacea is easy to distinguish from the pars muscularis due to its location in the dome of the diaphragm and its lower thickness. The layer of muscles can be recognized as a hypoechogenic plate, whereas – in the dome – the diaphragm appears as a fine echogenic line in the section image. The muscle plate of the diaphragm shortens and thickens during inspiration (Fig. 3.32). A distinct swelling of the diaphragmatic musculature can be observed now and again in patients with chronic obstructive diseases of the lung.

The diaphragmatic crura can be best depicted in longitudinal sections viewed laterally, on the left side through the retroperitoneum, and appear as moderately echogenic, elongated thread-like structures next to the spinal column. In a cross-section of the epigastric region, the diaphragmatic crura can be found next to the aorta and the inferior caval vein, directly above the origin of the celiac trunk coming out of the aorta. The extension of the diaphragmatic crura lateral of the trunk to caudal can differ individually.

Diaphragmatic hernias can be depicted sonographically, but not without difficulty. Therefore, when treating an adult, sonography is not the primary imaging method if there is a clinical suspicion. Hernias in infants and newborn babies can be detected by evidence of abdominal organs, e.g., stomach, intestines, liver, or spleen in the thorax (Fig. 3.33).

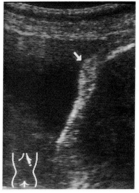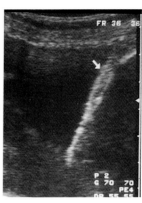

a
b

Fig. 3.32 a, b. Ultrasound image of the diaphragm with a pleural effusion, the transition from the muscular part to the thinner membranous part of the diaphragm in the dome is clearly demonstrable. During inspiration, the muscular part (**a**, *arrow*) shortens and thickens and relaxes during expiration (**b**, *arrow*)

Sonography is not a useful method for diagnosing the quite frequent axial hiatal hernias at the gastroesophageal junction. They can be distinguished endoscopically and the rugae of the stomach in the hernia can be depicted.

Ruptures of the diaphragm after a serious blunt abdominal trauma can also be recognized by a displacement of abdominal organs. In individual cases, the outline of the ruptures and the ensuing hiatus can be depicted during emergency sonographic examination of the abdomen. One should not be misled by an apparent diaphragmatic hiatus originating at an artifact corresponding to the outline shadow. The change in location of this hiatus with the changing position of the transducer is typical of this artifact.

In many cases, a – mostly sanguineous – pleural effusion resulting from an injury exists, which improves visibility into the thorax and makes the examination of the diaphragm easier. If the patient is seriously injured, an additional computed tomography is unavoidable in order to detect further thoracic or retroperitoneal injuries, which could not be depicted satisfactorily, if at all, sonographically.

Primary tumors of the diaphragm are very rare and are seldom diagnosed in the early stages of the disease; at best, they are an incidental finding (Fig. 3.34). Metastases in the diaphragm are also very rare; they can be the cause of unexplained

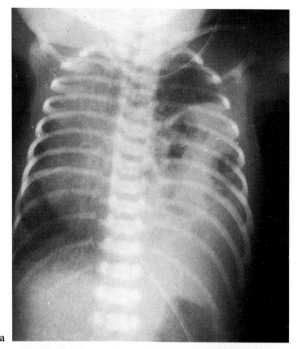

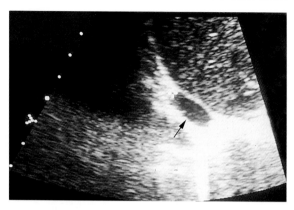

Fig. 3.34. Rare finding of a diaphragmatic lipoma. This was an incidental finding. The smoothly delineated tumor (*arrow*) presented similarly on computed tomography and showed fat density

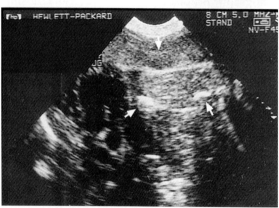

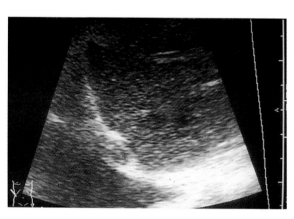

Fig. 3.33. **a** In the chest-X-ray of a newborn, air-containing intestinal organs in the left hemithorax are shown as a sign of a congenital diaphragmatic hernia on the left side. **b** Typical sonogram of the same newborn with a congenital diaphragmatic hernia on the left side with the stomach beneath the well distinguishable heart (*arrows*). Subxiphoidal cross section. (Images kindly provided by Prof. M. Teufel, Böblingen District Hospital, Germany)

Fig. 3.35. Sonomorphologically similar finding to that in Fig.3.30 in a patient with known bronchial carcinoma without any known metastasis up to that day. The finding was detected during a routine abdominal sonography. The finding was not comprehensible on computed tomography. An ultrasound-guided biopsy confirmed the clinical suspicion of metastasis of the known bronchogenic carcinoma

pain due to an infiltration of the adjacent nervous tissue (Fig. 3.35). In several cases, mainly in the context of metastatic breast cancer, the metastases could only be depicted using sonography, while in some cases they could be established on biopsy (Reuss J, unpublished data). Typical of metastases in the diaphragm is inclusion in the structure of the diaphragm. Metastases of the pleura and peritoneum are both positioned on the surface of the diaphragm. Large pleural metastases can grow deep into the diaphragm; they can even break through it, similar to pleural mesothelioma (Fig. 3.25).

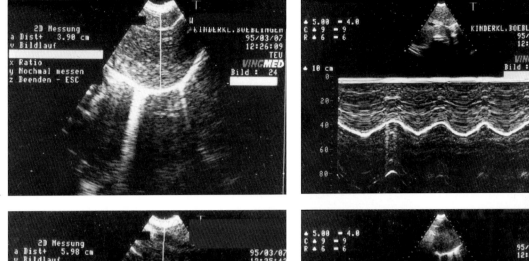

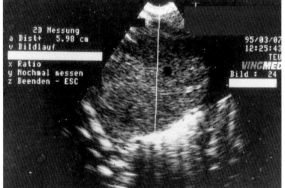

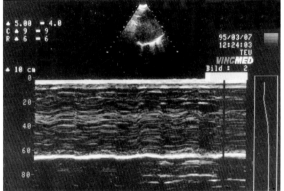

Fig. 3.36a–d. Traumatic paralysis of the diaphragm was suspected in a newborn infant. This suspicion was confirmed by a dynamic ultrasound examination on the right side. The finding was documented with a time–motion recording. a, b Healthy left side with definite rhythmic movements of the diaphragm, corresponding to the sinus curve-like line in the time–motion-recording. c, d Injured right side with the motionless diaphragm, corresponding to the almost straight line in the time–motion recording. (Images kindly provided by Prof. M. Teufel, Böblingen District Hospital, Germany)

The sonographic real-time examination is the most suitable method for a functional examination of the diaphragm. A normal, equilateral up and down of the diaphragm in harmony with respiration can be observed. Short video clips are optimal as documentation of diaphragmatic dysfunction. Paralysis of the diaphragm instantly attracts attention due to the absence of or paradoxical diaphragmatic movement. Pediatricians can document diaphragmatic paralysis following birth trauma without the need of X-ray examinations (Fig. 3.36). Sonography is very important in the process of clarifying a radiologically established, one-sided diaphragmatic eventration. Invasive thoracic or abdominal lesions with subsequent diaphragmatic eventration and absent respiratory movement are usually obvious due to their considerable extent. Apart from intra- and extra-organic tumors, excessive organ enlargement such as, e. g., a fatty liver or splenic enlargement due to, for example, a myeloproliferative disease can be causes for a diaphragmatic eventration. A subpulmonary effusion is frequently misinterpreted on chest X-ray as a double-sided diaphragmatic eventration. This can be easily recognized and further diagnosed sonographically. Other causes of a one-sided diaphragmatic eventration include subphrenic abscess or subphrenic encapsulated ascites, which can be depicted sonographically. The sonographic examination is unambiguous in these cases and hence no further imaging procedures are necessary.

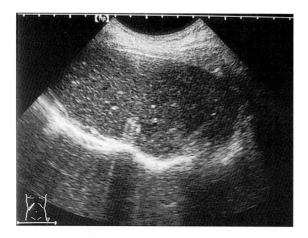

Fig. 3.37. Diaphragmatic fold. The ultrasound image clearly shows the doubling of the diaphragm in the liver. In a flat section under the diaphragm, this fold can be mistaken for a tumorous lesion in the liver

The diaphragmatic humps often observed on routine chest X-ray can also be imaged excellently on abdominal sonography. Rugae of the diaphragm which lead to crenation of the liver and less often of the spleen sometimes mimic focal lesions in these organs. An 'unfortunate' transverse section through such a diaphragmatic fissure might feign the existence of a target-like tumor. The relation becomes clear if longitudinal and transverse sections are taken. The doubling of the diaphragm can then also be depicted unambiguously (Fig. 3.37).

Summary

Despite the physical limitations of ultrasound, approximately 70% of the pleural surface can be accessed by sonography, especially from the costal and diaphragmatic aspects.

The normal parietal pleura can be visualized and delineated from circumscribed as well as diffuse pathological thickening. The normal visceral pleura is hidden by the total reflection at the surface of the aerated lung.

Sonographic evidence of a pleural effusion can be obtained from a diameter of 5 ml upwards. Ultrasound is much more sensitive than chest X-ray, especially with the patient in supine position; false-positive findings are not encountered. A more accurate estimation of the quantity of effusion can be made. Exudates are echogenic in one third of cases. Pleural thickening, nodular changes in the pleura, septa, and the formation of cavities occur only in cases of pleural exudates, whereas transudates are always anechoic.

Pleural metastases are characteristically hypoechoic and nodular–polypoid. Conclusions with regard to the primary tumor can be made only on the basis of histology. Pleural mesotheliomas can be delineated almost as clearly on sonography as on computed tomography, and the specificity of the former may be greater. Sonomorphological differentiation between mesothelioma, carcinosis and thickening may be difficult. Morphological and, in particular, functional diagnosis of the diaphragm by means of sonography is both reliable and convincing.

References

Baber CE, Hedlund LW, Oddson TA, Putman CE (1980) Differentiating empyemas and peripheral pulmonary abscess. Radiology 135:755–758

Bittner RC, Schnoy N, Schönfeld N et al. (1995) Hochauflösende Magnetresonanztomographie (HR-MRT) von Pleura und Thoraxwand: Normalbefund und pathologische Veränderungen. Fortschr Röntgenstr 162:296–303

Börner N (1986) Sonographische Diagnostik pleuropulmonaler Erkrankungen. Med Klinik 81:496–500

Börner N, Kelbel C, Lorenz J, Weilemann LS, Meyer J (1987) Sonographische Volumetrie und Drainage von Pleuraergüsen. Ultraschall Klein Prax 2:148–152

Collins JD, Burwell D, Furmanski S, Lorber P, Steckel RJ (1972) Minimal detectable pleural effusions. Radiology 105:51–53

Eibenberger KL, Dock WI, Ammann ME, Dorffner R, Hörmann MF, Grabenwöger F (1994) Quantification of pleural effusion: Sonography versus radiography. Radiology 191:681–684

Gehmacher O, Kopf A, Scheier M, Bitschnau R, Wertgen T, Mathis G (1997) Ist eine Pleuritis sonographisch darstellbar? Ultraschall in Med 18:214–219

Goecke W, Schwerk WB (1990) Die Real-Time-Sonographie in der Diagnostik von Pleuraergüssen. In: Gebhardt J, HackelöerB-J,v.Klinggräff G, Seitz K, ed., Ultraschalldiagnostik '89. Springer, Berlin Heidelberg New York, Tokio

Goerg C, Schwerk WB, Goerg K, Walters E (1991) Pleural effusion: an "acoustic window" for sonography of pleural metastasis. J Clin Ultrasound 19:93–97

Gryminski J, Krakówka P, Lypacewicz G (1976) The diagnosis of pleural effusion by ultrasonic and radiologic techniques. Chest 70:33–37

Joyner CR Jr, Herman RJ, Reid JM (1967) Reflected ultrasound in the detection and localization of pleural effusion. JAMA 200/5:(129–132)399–402

Kelbel C, Börner N, Schadmand S, Swars H, Weilemann LS (1990) Diagnostik von Pleuraergüssen bei intensivpflichtigen Patienten: Sonographie und Radiologie im Vergleich. In: Gebhardt J, Hackelöer BJ, v. Klinggräff G, Seitz K (ed), Ultraschalldiagnostik '89, Springer, Berlin, Heidelberg, New York, Tokio

Layer G, Schmitteckert H, Steudel A, Tuengerthal S, Schirren J, van Kaick G, Schild HH (1999) MRT, CT und Sonographie in der präoperativen Beurteilung der Primärtumorausdehnung beim malignen Pleuramesotheliom. Fortschr Röntgenstr 170:365–370

Loddenkemper R (1994) Pleuraerkrankungen. In: Ferlinz R, ed.: Pneumologie in Praxis und Klinik. Thieme, Stuttgart, New York, S 712–717

Lorenz J, Börner N, Nikolaus HP (1988) Sonographische Volumetrie von Pleuraergüssen. Ultraschall 9:212–215

Mowé G, Tellnes G (1995) Malignant pleural mesothelioma in Norway 1960–1992. Tidsskr Nor Laegeforen 115:706–709

Nakano N, Yasumitsu T, Kotake Y, Morino H, Ikezoe J (1994) Preoperativ histologic diagnosis of chest wall invasion by lung cancer using ultrasonically guided biopsy. J Thoracic Cardiovasc Surg 107:891–895

Reuss J (1996) Sonographic imaging of the pleura: nearly 30 years experience. Europ J Ultrasound 3:125–139

Ruffie P, Feld R, Minkin S, et al. (1989) Diffuse malignant mesothelioma of the in Ontario and Quebec: A retrospective study of 332 patients. J Clin Oncol 7:1157–1186

Sahn SA (1988) The pleura. Am Rev Respir Dis 138:184–234

Saito T, Kobayashi H, Kitamura S (1988) Ultrasonic appraoch to diagnosing chest wall tumors. Chest 94:1271–1275

Stark DD, Federle MP, Goodman PC, Podrsky AE, Webb WR (1983) Differentiating lung abscess and empyema: radiography and computed tomography. AJR 141:163–167

Sugarbaker DJ, Jaklitsch MT, Liptay MJ (1995) Mesothelioma and radical multimodality therapy: who benefits? Chest 107:345S–350S

Suzuki N, Saitoh T, Kitamura S (1993) Tumor invasion of the chest wall in lung cancer: diagnosis with US. Radiology 187:39–42

Theros EG, Feigin DS (1977) Pleural tumors and pulmonary tumors: differential diagnosis. Sem Roentgenol 12:239–247

Wu RG, Yuan A, Liauw YS, Chang DB, Yu CJ, Wu HD, Kuo SH, Luh KT, Yang PC (1994) Image comparison of real-time gray-scale ultrasound and color Doppler ultrasound for use in diagnosis of minimal pleural effusion. Am J Respir Crit care Med 150:510–514

Yang PC, Luh KT, Chang DB, Wu HD, Yu CJ, Kuo SH (1992) Value of sonography in determining the nature of pleural effusion: analysis of 320 cases. AJR 159:29–33

Yu CJ, Yang PC, Chang DB, Luh KT (1992) Diagnostic and therapeutic use of chest sonography: value in critically ill patients. AJR 159:695–701

4   Peripheral Lung Consolidation

4.1
Inflammatory Consolidations in the Lung: Pneumonia

G. MATHIS

Pathophysiological Prerequisites

In cases of lobular and segmental pneumonia, large amounts of air are displaced from the lung as a result of rich fibrinous exudation. Affected lobes or segments are depleted of air and sink in water. In the phase of engorgement and during hepatization, i. e., in the first week of disease, there are good conditions for pathological echo transmission. In this phase, pneumonia is imaged well on sonography. In the phase of lysis, the inflamed portion of the lung is ventilated to an increasing extent. Air reflexes superimpose deeper infiltrations. However, the sonographic image at this time underestimates the actual extent of disease. Focal pneumonias and interstitial pneumonias barely reach the pleura and are therefore not accessible to ultrasonographic imaging. However, bronchial pneumonias are often accompanied by involvement of the pleura and are therefore partly visualized by sonography.

Sonomorphology of Pneumonia

A number of sonomorphological criteria are characteristic of, but not specific for, pneumonic infiltrations. They are of varying intensity in the course of disease (Table 4.1).

Table 4.1. Sonomorphology of pneumonia

- Hepatoid in the early stage
- Homogeneous echoes
- Lenticular air trappings
- Blurred and serrated margins
- Air bronchogram
- Fluid bronchogram (poststenotic)
- Reverberation echoes in the margin
- Hypoechoic to anechoic in cases of abscesses (microabscesses!)

Engorgement Phase

In the initial phase of disease, i. e., in the engorgement phase, the pneumonic focus is hypoechoic, relatively homogeneous and hepatoid in nature. Its configuration is bizarre and it is rarely explicitly segmental like the pulmonary infarction or rounded like carcinomas and metastases. Its margins are irregular, serrated and somewhat blurred (Fig. 4.1).

Fluid Alveogram

In a densely subpleural location, one finds a broad and highly hypoechoic strip of varying extent and intensity (superficial fluid alveogram). Whether echogenic air bubbles are still visible or are seen again in a subpleural location depends on the extent and stage of disease (Targhetta et al. 1992; Kroegel and Reißig 2000).

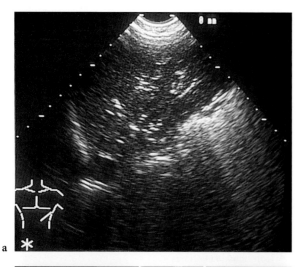

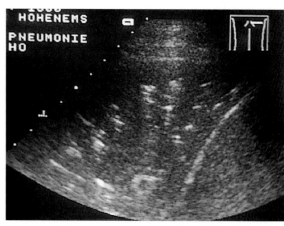

Fig. 4.2. Oblique section through a lobar pneumonia in the right lower lobe. Numerous lenticular air echoes extending nearly up to the pleura. The echo texture is very similar to that of the liver

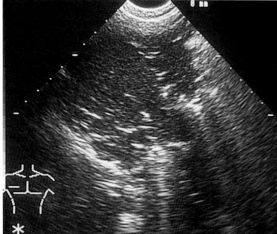

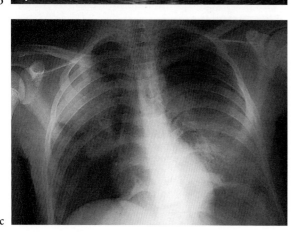

Fig. 4.3. Viral pneumonia with a small number of air trappings, homogeneously congested

Fig. 4.1a–c. A 22-year-old severely ill man with the clinical appearance of acute pneumonia. In the left lower lobe (**a**) and the right upper lobe (**b**), sonography shows liver-like infiltrations with air trappings and an air bronchogram. **c** Corresponding radiograph

Bronchial Aerogram

A marked bronchial aerogram (= bronchopneu-mogram, air bronchogram) with tree-like branches is seen in 87% of cases. The intense and long reflexes of the bronchial tree run between consolidated portions of the parenchyma. In all stages of pneumonia, the bronchial aerogram is more pronounced than in cases of pulmonary embolism. In some cases, one finds a small number of, but in most cases numerous, lenticular internal echoes no more than a few millimeters in size (Fig. 4.2). These echoes largely represent air, i.e., a partially imaged bronchial aerogram. These internal echoes can be partly explained by congested secretion of very different impedance (Mathis et al. 1990; Gehmacher et al. 1995). The air bronchogram visualized by sonography cannot be equated with that on a radiograph. Viral pneumonias are quite often more poorly ventilated and/or reveal less marked air bronchograms (Fig. 4.3).

Fluid Bronchogram

The fluid bronchogram is a further sonographic criterion of pneumonia. It is marked by anechoic tubular structures along the bronchial tree. The bronchial wall is echogenic and the fluid in the segmental bronchi are hypoechoic. The long reflexes around the bronchi are broader than those along vessel walls. Given good resolution, the bronchial walls are ribbed and vessel walls are smooth. Therefore, tubular structures can be easily classified on B mode images (Fig. 4.4). In cases of doubt, color-coded duplex sonography helps to distinguish between vessels and bronchi (Fig. 4.5). The fluid bronchogram can be seen in approximately 20% of patients with pneumonia and develops in the early phase of disease as a result of bronchial secretion or due to bronchial obstruction. A persistent fluid bronchogram always raises suspicion of poststenotic pneumonia and is an indication for bronchoscopic investigation. A tumor may be found or ruled out; the obstructive secretory embolus is aspirated, and material obtained for bacteriological investigation (Yang et al. 1992; Targhetta et al. 1992; Mathis 1996).

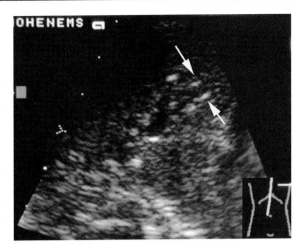

Fig. 4.4. Fluid bronchogram in the presence of poststenotic pneumonia. The bronchus can be delineated on the basis of broader reflexes compared to vessels; the bronchus is of varying wall thickness and ribbed

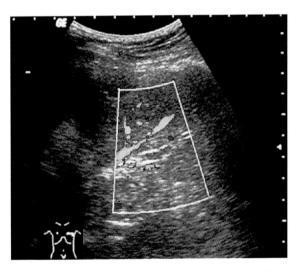

Fig. 4.5. Poststenotic pneumonia in the left upper lobe. Color-coded duplex sonography permits better identification of vessels. The reflex band of the bronchus is broader and interrupted

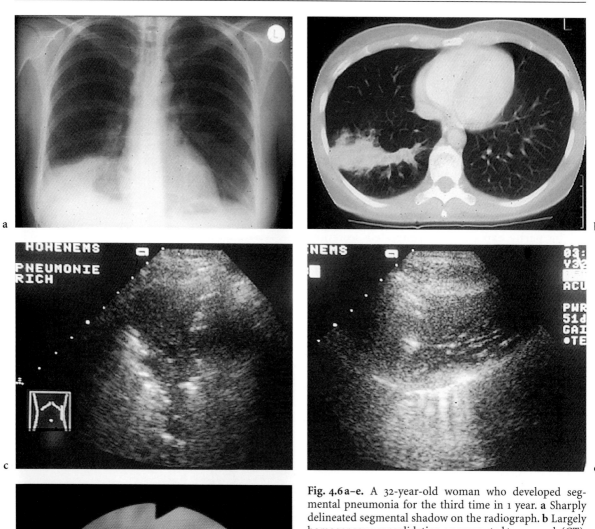

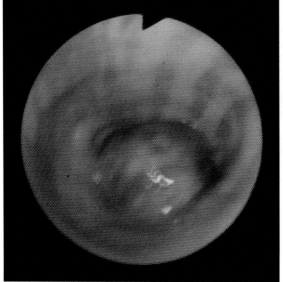

Fig. 4.6 a–e. A 32-year-old woman who developed segmental pneumonia for the third time in 1 year. **a** Sharply delineated segmental shadow on the radiograph. **b** Largely homogeneous consolidation on computed tomograph (CT). **c** On sonography, the form of the lesion is very similar to that on CT. The echotexture contains remarkably few air trappings. In the center, one finds a small anechoic area of fluid. **d** The longitudinal section reveals tubular structures; parallel to the vessel there is a typical fluid bronchogram. **e** Bronchoscopy confirms the adenocarcinoma, on surgery it is found to be in stage T1 N0

Poststenotic Pneumonia

Poststenotic pneumonias that develop in the periphery or margin of carcinomas are better delineated from the tumor by means of ultrasonography than radiography. Poststenotic pneumonia typically displays a fluid bronchogram (Fig. 4.6). Even for this condition, dynamic sonotomography is comparable with computed tomography (CT). Monitoring the effectiveness of therapy is important in this setting – is the pneumonia subsiding or is the tumor increasing in size (Braun et al. 1990; Yang et al. 1990)?

Circulation

On color-coded duplex sonography, pneumonia has a typical appearance: circulation is uniformly increased and branched, vessels have a normal course, but circulation is increased in the entire infiltrate up to beneath the pleura (Fig. 4.7). This is interesting when pneumonia needs to be differentiated from pulmonary infarctions that have poor or no blood flow, or even from tumors that have an irregular circulatory pattern. Carcinomas are strongly vascularized in their margins. Due to neovascularization, vessels in the margins of carcinomas have a characteristic corkscrew pattern (Gehmacher et al. 1995; Mathis 1996).

Abscess Formation

Bacterial pneumonias tend to fuse and form abscesses. This is the case in approximately 6% of patients with lobular pneumonia (this figure refers to radiographic investigations). Ultrasonography more commonly reveals *microabscesses* (Yang et al. 1991, 1992; Mathis 1996).
The *sonomorphology of pulmonary abscesses* is highly characteristic: Round or oval and largely anechoic foci (Fig. 4.8). Depending on the formation of a capsule, the margin is smooth, echodense, and white (Fig. 4.9). Blurred internal echoes are indicative of a high cell content or viscous pus rich

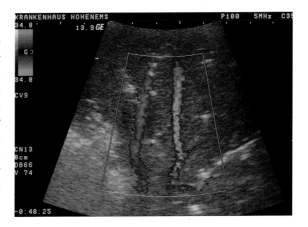

Fig. 4.7. On color-coded duplex sonography, pneumonias have an accentuated and regular pattern of circulation

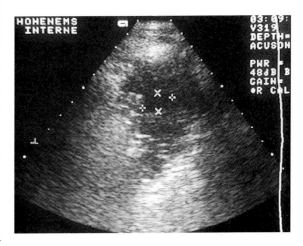

Fig. 4.8. On the 4th day of disease: microabscesses that could not be seen on radiographs. This abscess healed spontaneously

▶

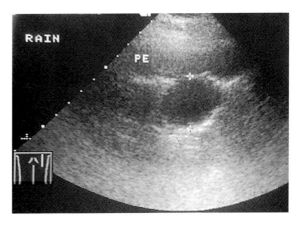

Fig. 4.9. Colliquative abscess in the phase of healing of pneumonia. The focus was emptied by ultrasound-guided needle aspiration; rapid healing followed. *PE*, pleural effusion

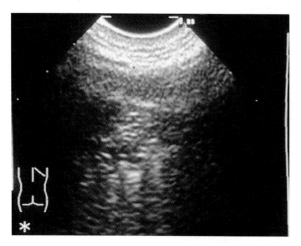

Fig. 4.10. Typical healing phase of bacterial pneumonia. The focus is receding, air trappings and reverberation artifacts are increasing

in protein. In cases of abscesses secondary to gas-forming pathogens, highly echogenic small air trappings move actively within the fluid in concordance with the respiratory rhythm. Septa are seen as echodense, fluttering threads. Artificial noise caused by the impedance difference between infiltrated parenchyma and abscess fluid is occasionally observed close to the head of the transducer. However, this should not be mistaken for internal echoes. Genuine internal echoes are always present in the depth of the image as well. In the early stage, small abscesses are seen as pathological collections of fluid and are found in an irregular anatomical location in the consolidated, liver-like infiltrate. Smooth margins and the echogenic capsule are absent. Microabscesses cannot be easily distinguished from vessels by means of color Doppler imaging.

Considering the moderate quantity of material for bacteriological investigation obtained from the sputum or from bronchial lavage, it is useful to obtain *a specimen for the detection of pathogens* by means of ultrasound-guided aspiration. When the puncture is performed with an ordinary injection needle, a thorough sonographic pre-investigation should be performed, if necessary under sonographic visual guidance, to ensure that air-filled lungs and vessels are avoided. The etiology of pulmonary infections can be determined by this method in 78 % of cases (Yang et al. 1992; Chen et al. 1993; Lee et al. 1993; Liaw et al. 1994; Mathis 1997).

Lung abscess drainage may be performed under sonographic or CT visual control. The selection of the instrument depends on the size of the lesion and the consistency of the contents of the abscess. Microabscesses measuring up to 2 cm in size can be punctured and emptied by ordinary aspiration. Large abscesses with thick viscous pus require large suction lavage drains, several types of which are commercially available. The position of the catheter is controlled by ultrasonography. The catheter is seen as a two-layered reflex (see Chap. 9, Fig. 9.7). The risk of a pneumothorax is minimized when one passes through the chest wall obliquely, in a regular fashion, and enters the lung at the site where the abscess is closest to the pleura. The risk of a dreaded bronchopleural fistula is minimized if a correct approach is used, i.e., when one traverses the homogeneous infiltrate and avoids ventilated areas (Yang et al. 1990; van Sonnenberg et al. 1991; Blank 1994; Mathis 1999).

Healing Phase

When pneumonia is in the healing phase, the infiltrated lung tissue is increasingly ventilated. Such air gives rise to reflection and reverberation artifacts. The pneumonia recedes on the ultrasonography image and appears smaller than on the chest radiograph (Figs. 4.10, 4.11).

The primary diagnosis of pneumonia is always based on clinical appearance and the chest radiograph, as the extent of infiltration is often underestimated on ultrasonography. Sonography is useful for monitoring the course of disease, especially in pregnant women and children (Schirg and Larbig 1999) (Table 4.2).

Table 4.2. Indications for sonography in the presence of pneumonia

- Pleural/basal shadow
- Imaging abscesses
- Identifying pathogens
- Abscess drainage
- Monitoring the course of disease

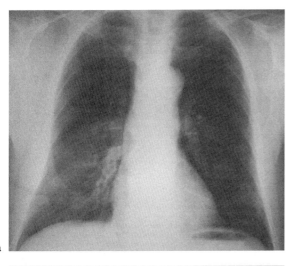

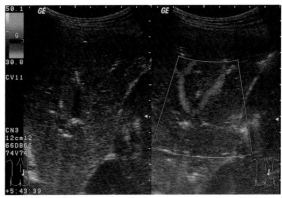

a

b

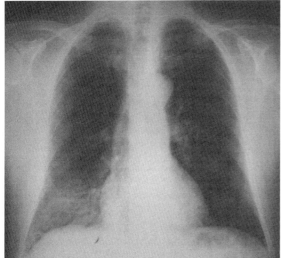

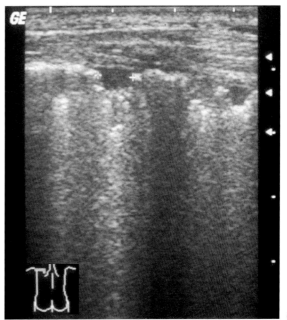

c

d

Fig. 4.11a–d. A 72-year-old man with clinically severe pneumococcus pneumonia. **a** Characteristic appearance on radiograph. **b** Sonography reveals, in terms of echostructure, a liver-like consolidation and a marked air bronchogram. After 1 week of antibiotic therapy, the patient is afebrile and healthy enough to be discharged. **c** The radiograph still clearly shows a marked residual infiltrate, while sonography only reveals small subpleural consolidations. **d** Subsequent sonographic controls are therefore of limited value and must at least be correlated with the clinical course of disease

▶

Fig. 4.12. Apical pulmonary tuberculosis with air trappings, whose extent is better seen here than on radiographs. Therefore, sonography was also suitable for monitoring the course of disease

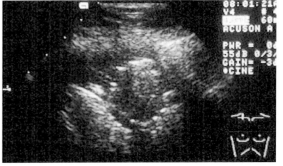

Tuberculosis

Lung tuberculosis has several features on the radiograph, and even more so on chest sonography. The value of sonography is, in general, not sufficiently researched. However, in certain settings, its value is beyond dispute. It can improve the detection of pathogens by means of ultrasound-guided aspiration or even biopsy and thus facilitate the imaging of subpleural colliquations and concomitant pleural fluid (Yuan et al. 1993; Kopf et al. 1994; Mathis 1996; Kregel and Reißig 2000).

Sonomorphology of Lung Tuberculosis

In cases of florid tuberculosis, a few or several hypoechoic lesions are seen (Figs. 4.12–4.14). Their appearance might be facilitated by a concomitant pleural effusion. They may be round or irregular in form and of relatively homogeneous texture. Depending on the size of the lesion, such infiltrates may also reveal air trappings as in pneumonia. Nodular spread in cases of miliary tuberculosis is imaged as multiple subpleural nodules a few millimeters in size (Fig. 4.15 a–e; Table 4.3).

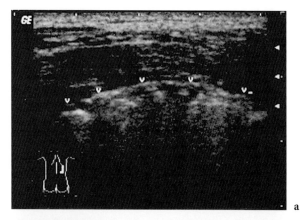

a

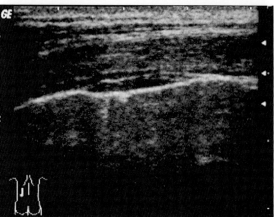

b

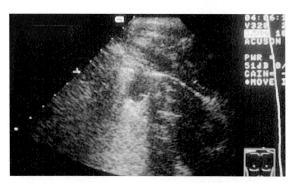

Fig. 4.13. Small tuberculotic focus at the apex of the lung. In this case, it was smaller on the sonographic image than on the radiograph

▶

Fig. 4.14 a–c. Miliary tuberculosis. **a** Fragmented pleura (>) with numerous subpleural nodules measuring 2–3 mm in size. **b** A 2-mm-broad focal pleural effusion that, of course, was not seen on the chest radiograph. **c** Chest radiograph: small speckled foci

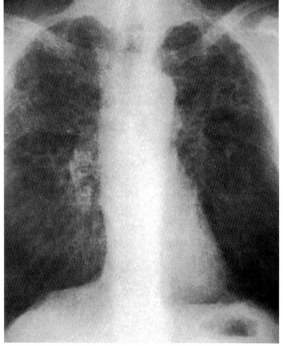

c

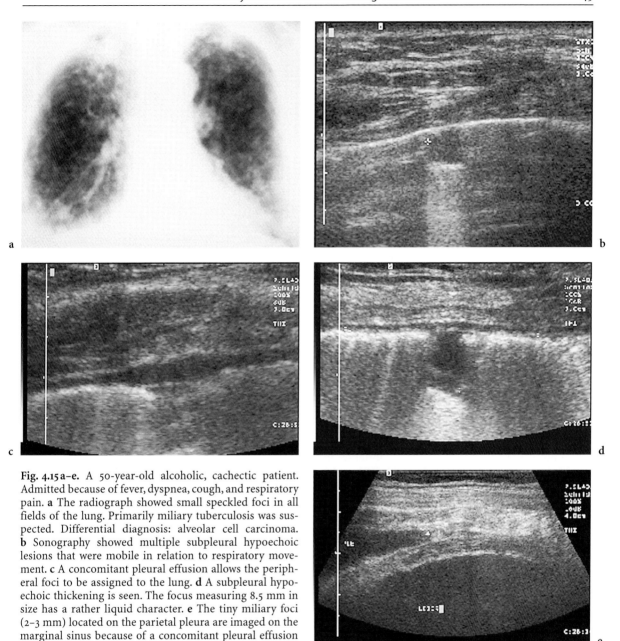

Fig. 4.15 a–e. A 50-year-old alcoholic, cachectic patient. Admitted because of fever, dyspnea, cough, and respiratory pain. **a** The radiograph showed small speckled foci in all fields of the lung. Primarily miliary tuberculosis was suspected. Differential diagnosis: alveolar cell carcinoma. **b** Sonography showed multiple subpleural hypoechoic lesions that were mobile in relation to respiratory movement. **c** A concomitant pleural effusion allows the peripheral foci to be assigned to the lung. **d** A subpleural hypoechoic thickening is seen. The focus measuring 8.5 mm in size has a rather liquid character. **e** The tiny miliary foci (2–3 mm) located on the parietal pleura are imaged on the marginal sinus because of a concomitant pleural effusion (*arrow*). The diagnosis of miliary tuberculosis is verified by ultrasonography-guided puncture of the liquid lesion

Table 4.3. Sonomorphology of pulmonary tuberculosis

- Pleural fluid
- Fragmentation of visceral pleura
- Subpleural infiltrations of various forms
- Air bronchogram in cases of larger infiltrations
- Broad reflection artifact in cavities

Colliquations can be imaged well, but air in cavities might be a disturbing factor and limit visualization. Even very small quantities of specific pleural effusion are seen. Pleural thickening may also be revealed. A patient's response to tuberculostatic therapy can be monitored well with sonography, especially in cases of pleural and subpleural tuberculotic lesions.

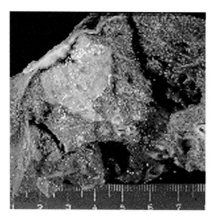
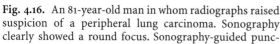
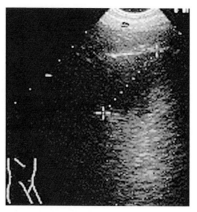

Fig. 4.16. An 81-year-old man in whom radiographs raised suspicion of a peripheral lung carcinoma. Sonography clearly showed a round focus. Sonography-guided punc-

ture revealed "no malignant cells." Interestingly, the band of visceral pleura was well preserved. Autopsy showed an old scarred tuberculoma

A "cold" *transmigrating abscess* is seen as a round, largely anechoic structure. When it is compressed, one finds floating marginal and internal echoes. Ultrasound-guided puncture will reveal acid-resisting rod bacteria (see Fig. 4.15e).

An old tuberculoma may raise suspicion of carcinoma on sonography as it does on radiographs, but rarely has "crow's feet" (Figs. 4.16, 4.17). Subpleural tuberculotic scars may be relatively echodense and star-shaped; in the presence of calcifications, they might reveal shadows.

The *value of sonography* in pulmonary tuberculosis lies in the detection of small pleural effusions that escape detection on radiographs. Such effusions can be punctured under ultrasound guidance in order to confirm the diagnosis. Even in cases of subpleural nodules, a diagnostic puncture is useful. When therapy is monitored, subpleural foci can be better followed on ultrasonography than on radiographs. However, ultrasound imaging of cavities is limited when air is present in the cavity. Chest radiographs and CT are indispensable in this setting.

In cases of more rare infectious, lung consolidations such as aspergillosis or *Echinococcus*, typical lesions can be imaged and important additional information (supplementing radiographs) obtained (Fig. 4.18).

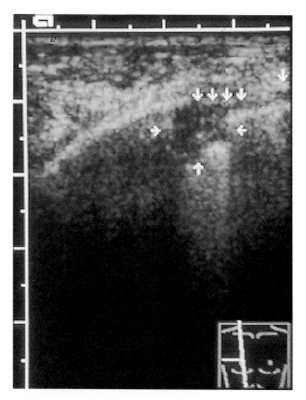

Fig. 4.17. Tuberculotic scars with small branches (*arrows*)

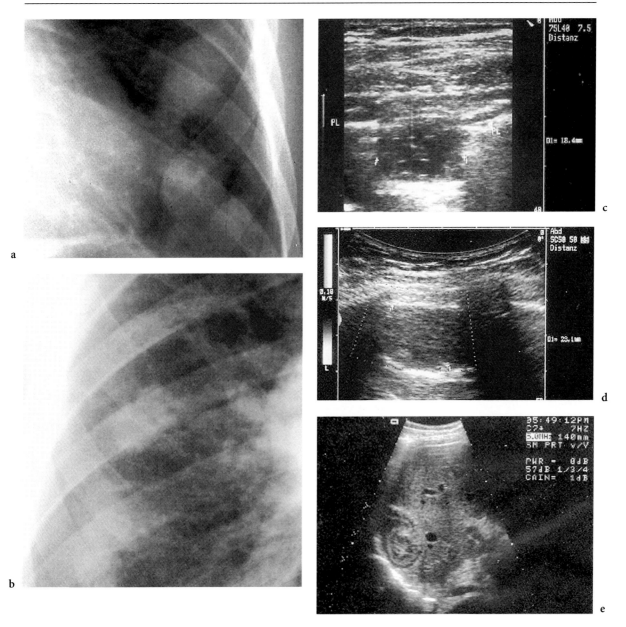

Fig. 4.18 a–e. *Echinococcus cysticus.* A 28-year-old man with a history of pulmonary *Echinococcus*. The patient was admitted to hospital with fever, cough, and marked dyspnea. **a, b** Radiographs revealed multiple round foci in the lung and pneumonic infiltrates. **c, d** Sonography showed round foci reaching the surface of the lung. Thick-walled cysts (*crosses*) with internal secondary cysts and no vascularization, on color Doppler sonography. Additionally, multiple areas indicative of pneumonia were identified. **e** *Echinococcus* was also found in the liver. Subsequent diagnostic procedures confirmed bilateral pneumonia – superinfection in the presence of preexisting pulmonary *Echinococcus*. The patient developed severe pulmonary hypertension in spite of antibiotic therapy and the administration of albendazole

Interstitial Lung Disease

Diseases of the framework lung cannot be imaged by sonography. In fact, in this setting, sonography is nearly meaningless as a primary diagnostic tool. However, it was shown that such diseases are frequently accompanied by *involvement of the pleura* and the latter is better imaged by sonography than by other imaging procedures (Figs. 4.19). Here, the value of sonography lies in the detection of minimal pleural effusions and subpleural infiltrations. Both can be punctured for the purpose of diagnosis and then monitored during therapy (Kroegel and Reißig 2000; Wohlgenannt et al. 2000).

Summary

The sonomorphology of pneumonic lung infiltrations reveals typical changes (bronchoaerograms, colliquations, parapneumonic effusions). The extent of infiltration is frequently underestimated due to artifacts on ultrasonography. The value of chest sonography in this setting is not in the realm of primary diagnosis, but in the estimation of accompanying pleural fluid, in the timely detection of abscesses, in the ultrasound-guided obtaining of pathogens, in abscess drainage, and occasionally also in monitoring the course of disease, especially in children.

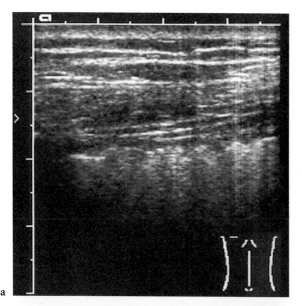

a

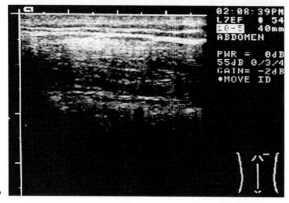

b

Fig. 4.19 a, b. Female patient with a farmer's lung: Sonography shows minimal pleural effusions, fragmentation of the visceral pleura and minimal subpleural consolidations

References

Anzböck W, Braun U, Stellamor K (1990) Pulmonale und pleurale Raumforderungen in der Sonographie. In: Gebhardt J, Hackelöer BJ, Klingräff v. G, Seitz K (Hrsg) Ultraschalldiagnostik '89. Springer, Berlin Heidelberg New York Tokyo, S 394–396

Blank W (1994) Sonographisch gesteuerte Punktionen und Drainagen. In: Braun B, Günther R, Schwerk WB (Hrsg) Ultraschalldiagnostik Lehrbuch und Atlas. ecomed, Landsberg/Lech III-11.1:15–22

Braun U, Anzböck W, Stellamor K (1990) Das Sonographische Erscheinungsbild der Pneumonie. In: Gebhardt J, Hackelöer BJ, Klingräff G v, Seitz K et al. (Hrsg) Ultraschalldiagnostik '89. Springer, Berlin Heidelberg New York Tokyo, S 392–393

Chen CH, Kuo ML, Shih JF, Chang TP, Perng RP (1993) Etiologic diagnosis of pulmonary infection by ulrasonically guided percutaneous lung aspiration. Chung Hua Taiwan 51:5

Gehmacher O, Mathis G, Kopf A, Scheier M (1995) Ultrasound imaging of pneumonia. Ultrasound Med Biol 21:1119–1122

Gehmacher O (1996) Ultrasound pictures of pneumonia. Eur J Ultrasound 3:161–167

Kopf A, Metzler J, Mathis G (1994) Sonographie bei Lungentuberkulose. Bildgebung 61:S2:12

Kroegel C, Reißig A (2000) Transthorakale Sonographie. Thieme, Stuttgart

Lee LN, Yang PC, Kuo SH, Luh KT, Chang DB, Yu CJ (1993) Diagnosis of pulmonary cryptococcosis by ultrasound guided perdutaneous aspiration. Thorax 48:75–78

Liaw YS, Yang PC et al. (1994) The bacteriology of obstructive pneumonitis. Am J Respir Crit Care Med 149: 1648–1653

Mathis G, Metzler J Fußenegger D, Feurstein M, Sutterlütti G (1992) Ultraschallbefunde bei Pneumonie. Ultraschall Klin Prax 7:45–49

Mathis G (1996) Lungen- und Pleurasonographie. 2. Aufl., Springer, Berlin Heidelberg New York Tokyo, pp 81–85

Mathis G (1997) Thoraxsonography – Part II: Peripheral pulmonary consolidation. Ultrasound Med Biol 23: 1141–1153

Mathis G, Bitschnau R, Gehmacher O, Dirschmid K (1999) Ultraschallgeführte transthorakale Punktion. Ultraschall Med 20:226–235

Targhetta R, Chavagneux R, Bourgeois JM, Dauzat M, Balmes P, Pourcelot L (1992) Sonographic approach to diagnosing pulmonary consolidation. J Ultrasound Med 11:667–672

Schirg E, Larbig M (1999) Wert des Ultraschalls bei der Diagnostik kindlicher Pneumonien. Ultraschall Med 20: S34

van Sonnenberg E, Agostino H, Casola G, Wittich GR, Varney RR, Harker C (1991) Lung abscess: CT-guided drainage. Radiology 178:347–351

Weinberg B, Diaboumakis EE, Kass EG, Seife B, Zvi ZB (1986) The air bronchogram: sonographic demonstration. AJR 147:593–595

Wohlgenannt S, Gehmacher O, Mathis G (2001) Thoraxsonographische Veränderungen bei interstitiellen Lungenerkrankungen. Ultraschall Med, in press

Yang PC, Lee YC, Wu HD, Luh KT (1990) Lung tumors associated with obstructive pneumonitis: US studies. Radiology 174:593–595

Yang PC, Luh KT, Lee YC (1991) Lung abscesses: ultrasonography and ultrasound-guided transthoracic aspiration. Radiology 180:171–175

Yang PC, Luh KT, Chang DB, Yu CJ, Kuo SH, Wu HD (1992) Ultrasonographic evaluation of pulmonary consolidation. Am Rev Resp Dis 146:757–762

Yu CJ, Yang PC, Wu HD, Chang DB, Kuo SH, Luh KT (1993) Ultrasound study in unilateral hemithorax opification. Am Rev Respir Dis 147:430–434

Yuan A, Yang PC, Chang DB et al. (1993) Ultrasound guided aspiration biopsy for pulmonary tuberculosis with unusual radiographic appearances. Thorax 48:167–170

4.2
Neoplastic Consolidations in the Lung: Primary Lung Tumors and Metastases

S. BECKH

In diagnostic imaging of malignant pulmonary foci, sonography is a valuable adjunct to sectional images obtained by radiological procedures (Stender et al. 1994; Müller 1997; Fraser et al. 1999). Thanks to its high resolution, the ultrasonography image yields very important additional information. For instance, vessels can be imaged without contrast medium (Civardi et al. 1993; Yang 1996; Hsu et al. 1998).

Lung consolidations can only be documented on sonography when no aerated tissue hinders echo transmission. In terms of staging and treatment planning in cases of malignant pulmonary disease, procedures that yield sectional images, e.g., CT and magnetic resonance tomography, are absolutely essential in order to obtain an overview of the entire thorax (Wunderbaldinger et al. 1999). As a rule, sonography is performed when the entire range of radiographic findings are known.

In the diagnosis of lung carcinoma, the specific questions raised during sonographic investigation are as follows:

- Criteria to determine the benign or malignant nature of disease
- Imaging guidance for biopsy
- Whether surgery and resection can be performed
- Controls to monitor therapy
- Imaging vascular complications (inflow congestion, thrombosis)
- Detecting lymph node metastases

Pulmonary malignancies may have a highly variable *echotexture*. They are usually hypoechoic, moderately echodense, or very inhomogeneously structured; more rarely, they are nearly anechoic (Mathis 1997; Mathis et al. 1999; Table 4.4). However, the echotexture alone does not permit the investigator to decide whether the disease is malignant or benign (Figs. 4.20, 4.21).

In contrast to acute inflammatory infiltrations, the sonomorphology of malignant foci does not change during a short course of disease. Chronic carnifying pneumonia and peripheral callused cicatricial foci are problematic in terms of differential diagnosis. In particular, it is difficult to differentiate these entities from malignant disease (Mathis 1997).

Decisive criteria to grade the malignant or benign nature of a pulmonary focus are as follows:

- *Contours* of the lung surface
- *Margins* to ventilated lung tissue
- *Infiltration* of adjacent structures of the chest wall
- *Destruction* of normal tissue architecture
- *Displacement* of regular vessels
- *Neovascularization*

The *contours* of the lung surface are especially well delineated against the surrounding pleural fluid. Figure 4.22 shows the uneven polypoid surface of an adenocarcinoma in the left upper lobe.

A benign inflammatory infiltration would never lead to such a tuberous deformation of the lung surface.

Malignant foci frequently have very *sharp margins* towards lung tissue (Fig. 4.23), but may occasionally have *fringed or finger-shaped ramifications* into the normally ventilated parenchyma – a sign of invasive growth (Fig. 4.24).

Table 4.4. Sonomorphology of pulmonary carcinomas

Form	Echotexture	Vessels	Complex structures
Sharp margins	Inhomogeneous	Displacement of vessels	Residual ventilated areas
Rounded	Hypoechoic	Destruction of vessels	Concomitant pneumonia in the margin
Polypoid	Rarely echogenic	Neovascularization	Solid space-occupying mass/pneumonia
Ramifications	Rarely anechoic	–	Bacterial/mycotic colonization
Serrated margins	–	–	Bizarre pattern, large necroses

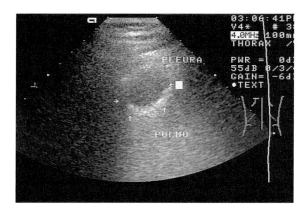

Fig. 4.20. On the left side, in dorsal location, between the scapula and the vertebral column, a hypoechoic circular focus (*arrows*) sharply delineated against ventilated lung tissue; thickened pleura (+ – +, 7.8 mm). Histological investigation of the specimen from the upper lobe revealed squamous cell carcinoma

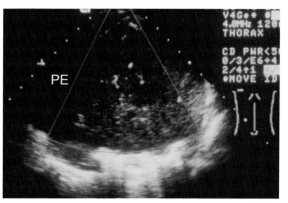

Fig. 4.22. In the left upper lobe, sonography showed a large tumor with a cauliflower-like surface, surrounded by pleural effusion (*PE*). In the margin of the tumor, there are numerous tortuous vessels. Sonography-guided biopsy: poorly differentiated adenocarcinoma

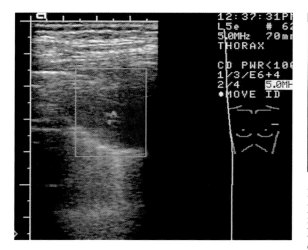

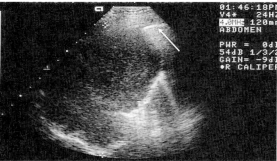

Fig. 4.23. Large hypoechoic space-occupying mass with polycyclic margins in the right upper lobe, with its maximum medial dimensions extending into the mid axillary line. The broad base of the tumor lies adjacent to the parietal pleura. Caudally, an unremarkable echogenic pleural line (*arrow*). Sonography-guided biopsy: poorly differentiated, solid-growing, nonkeratinizing squamous cell carcinoma

Fig. 4.21. A 40-year-old man with recurrent eosinophilic pleural effusions. Radiography showed a peripheral focus in the left upper lobe. In the anterior axillary line, in the 2nd intercostal space, sonography showed a relatively sharply margined hypoechoic peripheral pulmonary focus with central vessels. Thoracoscopic removal of the lesion revealed the diagnosis of hyalinosis and callus formation. The source of the pleural effusions is still unclear

▶

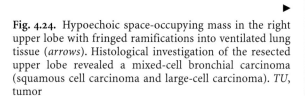

Fig. 4.24. Hypoechoic space-occupying mass in the right upper lobe with fringed ramifications into ventilated lung tissue (*arrows*). Histological investigation of the resected upper lobe revealed a mixed-cell bronchial carcinoma (squamous cell carcinoma and large-cell carcinoma). *TU*, tumor

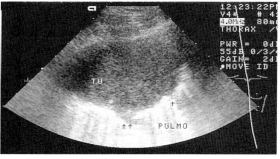

In contrast to inflammatory foci, such solid malignant formations in marginal zones are not ventilated and are therefore more sharply demarcated against the surrounding tissue.

Almost at first glance, a malignancy *invading* adjacent structures is indicative of the aggressive nature of the tumor (Suzuki et al. 1993). In the case of a Pancoast tumor, penetration of a space-occupying mass through the dome of the pleura can be clearly imaged (Fig. 4.25).

Malignant invasion of the chest wall frequently causes local pain. Targeted investigation of the region with the transducer will help to diagnose the condition early (Fig. 4.26).

Invasion into adjacent structures of the chest wall is a very reliable sign of malignant growth. In terms of differential diagnosis only one disease is likely to be present here, namely actinomycosis or nocardiosis (Corrin 1999; Fig. 4.27).

The inflammation frequently spreads into the chest wall. Regular cardinal anatomic structures of the lung, however, are well preserved within the pneumonic infiltration of tissue. In conjunction with clinical symptoms and bacteriological investigation they permit the investigator to make the correct diagnosis.

Malignant invasion *destroys* the normal texture of tissue. Bronchial branches may be displaced or fully destroyed (Fig. 4.28).

The original normal vessels will be displaced (Fig. 4.29) or will disappear altogether (Fig. 4.28).

In some cases, vessels of the tumor itself will be found, especially in the margin (see Fig. 4.22). Such vessels display a tortuous course (Yuan et al. 1994; Mathis 1997; Hsu et al. 1996, 1998).

For further planning of treatment in terms of *whether the entity can be operated on and resected*, a detailed dynamic investigation has to be performed. In order to decide between video-assisted thoracoscopy (VATS) and thoracotomy, it is important to know whether the pathological entity is widely fixed to the parietal pleura or is freely movable with the lung (Landreneau et al. 1998). However, adherence alone does not permit the investigator to determine whether a finding is malignant or benign.

In the course of tumor staging, it is important to perform sonographic investigations of accessible lymph node regions (Sugama and Kitamura 1992), and the vena cava with its afferent vessels (Ko et al. 1994; Fig. 4.30).

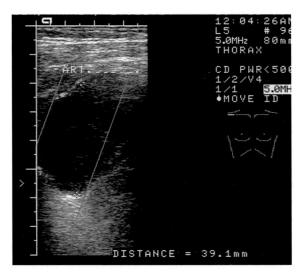

Fig. 4.25. A 55-year-old woman with pain radiating into the shoulder and right arm. The probe placed in supraclavicular location on the right side showed a tumor penetrating the dome of the pleura and invading muscular portions of the chest wall. In the upper portion of the tumor, there is a strong vessel. Sonography-guided biopsy: poorly differentiated adenocarcinoma. *ART*, artery

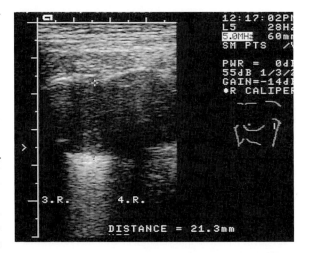

Fig. 4.26. The (female) patient had fallen down stairs 6 months previously and had been having renewed pain on the left side of the chest for 4 weeks. Computed tomography raised suspicion of a hematoma. Sonography showed a space-occupying mass that infiltrated the musculature of the chest wall. Circumscribed destruction of the lateral aspect of the 3rd and 4th rib. Sonography-guided biopsy: poorly differentiated adenocarcinoma

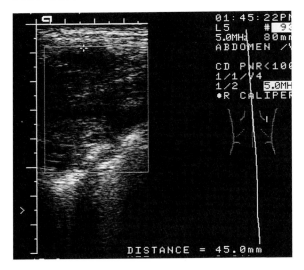

Fig. 4.27. This severely ill 37-year-old man had high fever and dyspnea. Radiographs showed extensive infiltration of the right lower lobe, continuing into the chest wall. Sonography clearly revealed the focus extending beyond the margins; it also demonstrated well preserved, regular bronchial branches and vessels. Therefore, in spite of the extensive nature of the lesion, a malignancy appeared very unlikely. In a surgically obtained biopsy specimen, actinomyces were found. Treatment with high-dose penicillin caused the invasion to regress within 10 weeks to a narrow, basal callus

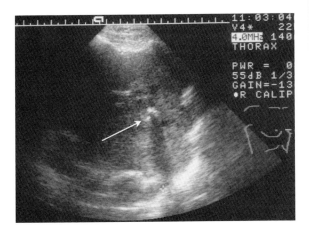

Fig. 4.28. A 50-year-old man with retrosternal pain that initially raised suspicion of coronary heart disease. Sonography showed a large tumor in the left upper lobe, in parasternal location, penetrating the mediastinum, and complete destruction of bronchial branches. Calcification and dorsal echo obliteration (*arrow*) within the tumor. Sonographic biopsy. Poorly differentiated adenocarcinoma with tumor cell complexes in lymphatic spaces

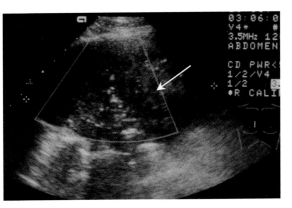

Fig. 4.29. After resection of the upper lobe on the right side 5 years previously due to an adenocarcinoma, the patient had a hypoechoic focus in the right upper field, with partially ventilated areas and a markedly curved displacement of a large vascular branch (*arrow*). Sonographic biopsy: renewed adenocarcinoma

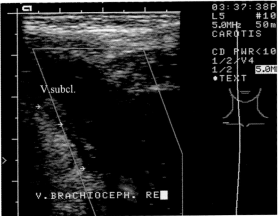

Fig. 4.30. This 69-year-old man with known adenocarcinoma on the right side and mediastinal lymphomas developed a swelling in the right arm. Sonography from a supraclavicular approach on the right side showed recent thrombosis of the subclavian vein

The assessment of malignant foci might be rendered difficult by their very *heterogeneous structural pattern* (Pan et al. 1993; see Table 4.4).

Tumor consolidations may still contain residually ventilated bronchial branches (see Fig. 4.29) or *colliquations* and/or *necrotic zones* (Fig. 4.31).

Lung tissue adjacent to a tumor might be affected by inflammation (Fig. 4.32) or contain calcifications (Fig. 4.28).

In a diseased portion of the lung, solid portions of the tumor might exist along with complex inflammatory infiltrations (Fig. 4.33).

Sonographic assessment of bronchoalveolar carcinoma is highly problematic. On the one hand multiple peripheral consolidations with variable air content might mimic multifocal pneumonia (Fig. 4.34). On the other hand one may only find an uncharacteristic uneven lung surface (Fig. 4.35).

In all cases of indefinite pulmonary foci, sonography may serve as an important aid. It helps the investigator to decide on the subsequent diagnostic procedure – either immediately in terms of a sonography-assisted biopsy (Greenspan and Sostman 1994; Mathis et al. 1999) or as a complementary imaging method to select the appropriate surgical procedure.

Pulmonary metastases are documented on sonography when they reach the margin of the lung. Due to poor visibility in this region, ultrasound is not a suitable screening method. Metastases have no small air trappings and are usually homogeneously hypoechoic; occasionally, they have branches extending into tissue (Mathis et al. 1999). Pathological vessels are predominantly found in the margin (Table 4.5; Fig. 4.36).

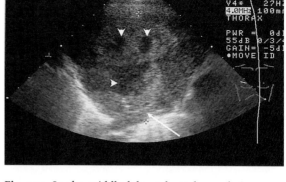

Fig. 4.31. In the middle lobe, a large hypoechoic space-occupying mass with dorsomedially invasive, residually ventilated parts (*arrow*) and several necrotic areas in the central portion (*tips of arrows*). Sonographic biopsy: well to moderately differentiated keratinizing squamous cell carcinoma

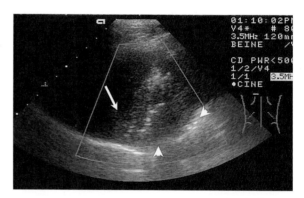

Fig. 4.32. In the left upper lobe in dorsal paravertebral location, a hypoechoic space-occupying mass, rather sharp lateral margins (*arrow*), an invasively inflamed area (*tips of arrows*) adjacent to it in the medial aspect. Clinically, the patient initially had marked signs of inflammation. Under antibiotic therapy, the invasive pneumonic entity resolved. A sonographic biopsy from solid portions of the tumor revealed a poorly differentiated adenocarcinoma

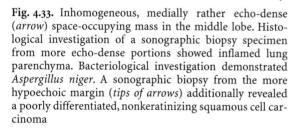

Fig. 4.33. Inhomogeneous, medially rather echo-dense (*arrow*) space-occupying mass in the middle lobe. Histological investigation of a sonographic biopsy specimen from more echo-dense portions showed inflamed lung parenchyma. Bacteriological investigation demonstrated *Aspergillus niger*. A sonographic biopsy from the more hypoechoic margin (*tips of arrows*) additionally revealed a poorly differentiated, nonkeratinizing squamous cell carcinoma

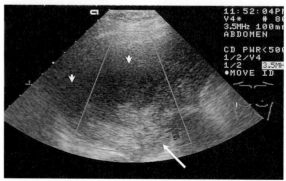

Table 4.5. Sonomorphology of pulmonary metastases

Form	Echotexture	Vessels
Round	Hypoechoic	Bizarre new formation of vessels in the margin
Oval	No ventilated areas	–
Serrated	Necrosis possible	–
Sharp margins	–	–

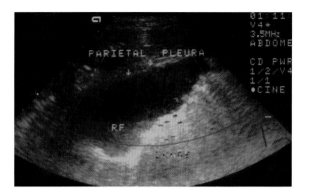

Fig. 4.36. Six months before the patient was admitted to hospital, a malignant fibrous histiocytoma of the skull had been resected. In the meantime, a new focus had developed in the right upper lobe. Investigation of sputum showed acid-resistant rod bacteria. Sonography revealed a homogeneous hypoechoic space-occupying mass with ramifications in the ventilated lung and tortuous vessels in the margins. Based on sonomorphology alone these findings could not be interpreted as a tuberculotic inflammation, but were more likely indicative of a solid tumor. Sonographic biopsy confirmed the suspected diagnosis of metastasis of the malignant fibrous histiocytoma

Sonographic images were digitized and recorded with the ClinicWinData system (E & L Computer Systeme, Erlangen, Germany).

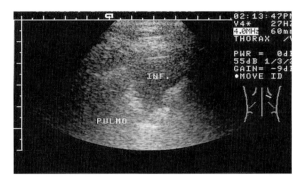

Fig. 4.34. In the right upper lobe, dorsally, a nearly triangular invasive focus with blurred margins. Thoracoscopic biopsy confirmed a bronchoalveolar carcinoma. *INF*, infiltration; *PULMO*, lung

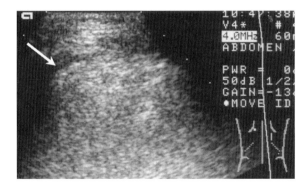

Fig. 4.35. This patient had a bronchoalveolar carcinoma confirmed by radiographic investigation and bronchoscopic biopsy. The carcinoma filled the entire lower lobe on the right side. Sonography only showed an irregular, finely grained lung surface (*arrow*)

Summary

Sonography does not permit the investigator to make a distinction between metastases and peripheral carcinoma. The interpretation must take the patient's medical history and survey radiographs into account. In terms of differential diagnosis, the formation of foci in the parietal pleura must be excluded by dynamic investigation. Even benign pulmonary foci, e.g., hamartoma or hemangiofibroma, might extend up to the periphery of the lung as hypoechoic formations. Cyst walls may be of varying thickness. They usually have an anechoic content. Occasionally, they contain fluid with internal echoes. In order to differentiate between a cyst and a pulmonary abscess or an encapsulated empyema, the diagnostic procedure must take clinical parameters and CT investigations into account. In the final analysis, bacteriological, cytological, and histological investigations are of decisive importance.

References

Civardi G, Fornari F, Cavanna L et al. (1993) Vascular signals from pleura-based lung lesions studied with pulsed Doppler ultrasonography. J Clin Ultrasound 21: 617–622

Corrin B (1999) Actinomycosis. In: Corrin B (ed) Pathology of the Lungs. Churchill Livingstone, London, S 194–195

Fraser RS, Müller NL, Colman N, Paré PD (1999) Fraser and Paré's diagnosis of diseases of the chest. Saunders, Philadelphia, S 299–338

Greenspan RH, Sostman HD (1994) Radiographic Techniques. In: Murray JF, Nadel JA (eds) Textbook of respiratory medicine. Saunders, Philadelphia, S 638–644

Hsu WH, Ikezoe J, Chen CY et al. (1996) Color Doppler ultrasound signals of thoracic lesions. Am J Respir Crit Care Med 153:1938–1951

Hsu WH, Chiang CD, Chen CY et al. (1998) Color Doppler ultrasound pulsatile flow signals of thoracic lesions: comparison of lung cancers and benign lesions. Ultrasound Med Biol 24:1087–1095

Ko JC, Yang PC, Yuan A et al. (1994) Superior vena cava syndrome. Am J Respir Crit Care Med 149:783–787

Landreneau RJ, Mack MJ, Dowling RD et al. (1998) The role of thoracoscopy in lung cancer management. Chest 113:6S–12S

Mathis G (1997) Thoraxsonography – Part II: Peripheral pulmonary consolidation. Ultrasound Med Biol 23:1141–1153

Mathis G, Bitschnau R, Gehmacher O et al. (1999) Ultraschallgeführte transthorakale Punktion. Ultraschall Med 20:226–235

Müller W (1997) Ultraschall-Diagnostik. In: Rühle KH (Hrsg) Pleura-Erkrankungen. Kohlhammer, Stuttgart, S 31–44

Pan JF, Yang PC, Chang DB et al. (1993) Needle aspiration biopsy of malignant lung masses with necrotic centers. Chest 103:1452–1456

Stender HS, Majewski A, Schober O et al. (1994) Bildgebende Verfahren in der Pneumologie. In: Ferlinz R (Hrsg) Pneumologie in Praxis und Klinik. Thieme, Stuttgart, S 176–178

Sugama Y, Kitamura S (1992) Ultrasonographic evaluation of neck and supraclavicular lymph nodes metastasized from lung cancer. Internal Medicine 31:160–164

Suzuki N, Saitoh T, Kitamura S et al. (1993) Tumor invasion of the chest wall in lung cancer: diagnosis with US. Radiology 187:39–42

Yang PC (1996) Review paper: Color Doppler ultrasound of pulmonary consolidation. Eur J Ultrasound 3:169–178

Yuan A, Chang DB, Yu CJ et al. (1994) Color Doppler sonography of benign and malignant pulmonary masses. AJR 163:545–549

Wunderbaldinger P, Bankier AA, Strasser G et al. (1999) Staging des Bronchialkarzinoms. Radiologe 39:525–537

4.3
Vascular Lung Consolidations: Pulmonary Embolism and Pulmonary Infarction

G. Mathis

Pulmonary embolism is the most frequently clinically undiagnosed cause of death. Autopsy observations have shown a frequency of 10%–15%. In cases of chronic heart failure, the rate is as high as 30%. Again, pulmonary embolism is the cause of death in 40% of these. A total of 10% of deaths in hospitals are caused by pulmonary embolism. In a further 10%, pulmonary embolism is involved in a causal way. As the clinical symptoms are nonspecific and the chest radiograph is not sensitive, the most important diagnostic step is still to consider the possibility of pulmonary embolism in the first place (Table 4.6). The clinician is called upon to apply every method that will improve the diagnosis of pulmonary embolism.

Pathophysiological Prerequisites for Ultrasound Imaging of Pulmonary Embolism

A few minutes after a secondary pulmonary artery is occluded, the surfactant collapses. Interstitial fluid and erythrocytes flow into the alveolar space. Hemorrhagic congestion offers ideal conditions for ultrasound imaging. These consolidations are oriented towards the pleura. They are open at the periphery along with their base, which creates good conditions for transthoracic sonography (Joyner et al. 1966; Miller et al. 1967; Mathis and Dirschmid 1993; Table 4.7).

The pulmonary embolism is a dynamic process. Small hemorrhages are rapidly absorbed by local fibrinolysis, as the intimal layer of pulmonary arteries has a substantial fibrinolytic capacity. Massive or fulminant pulmonary embolism is often preceded by small premonitory embolism which, when detected on time, cause appropriate therapeutic measures to be initiated.

The *classic pulmonary infarction* has two prerequisites: an embolic closure of small branches of pulmonary arteries and a preexisting congestion of blood in the minor circulation. The latter prerequisite is definitely no longer valid, as pulmonary infarctions are often found to occur in young patients with an entirely healthy cardiac system. When a larger pulmonary artery is occluded, compensatory blood supply is ensured via precapillary bronchopulmonary anastomoses, so that an infarction rarely occurs.

The frequency of *hemorrhagic pulmonary infarction* in cases of pulmonary embolism is reported to range between 25% and 60%. According to recent studies, however, the rate is much higher. This was proven by new imaging procedures that were previously not available. What pathologists described in the 1960s can be imaged today with sonography and CT. The dynamics of change from the early infarction which can become reperfused up to the stage of pronounced tissue necrosis can be documented sonographically in a water bath and subsequently confirmed in terms of pathology, anatomy, and even histology (Könn and Scheijbal 1978; Hartung 1984, Heath and Smith 1988; Lammers and Bloor 1988; Mathis and Dirschmid 1993).

Table 4.6. Clinical diagnosis in cases of pulmonary embolism established as the cause of death by autopsy

Author	Year	Patients	Accuracy
Morgentaler and Ryu	1995	92	32%
Morpurgo and Schmid	1995	92	28%

Table 4.7. Pathophysiological prerequisites for ultrasonographic imaging in cases of pulmonary embolism

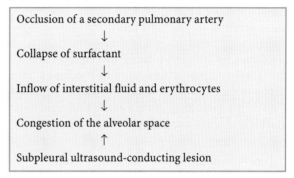

Occlusion of a secondary pulmonary artery
↓
Collapse of surfactant
↓
Inflow of interstitial fluid and erythrocytes
↓
Congestion of the alveolar space
↑
Subpleural ultrasound-conducting lesion

Sonomorphology of Pulmonary Infarction

Early Pulmonary Infarctions

Early pulmonary infarctions that can be reperfused are visualized as homogeneous structures with a pleural base that is occasionally somewhat protruded. The lesion is relatively homogeneous and hypoechoic. The margin is fairly indistinct in the first few hours, but is otherwise smoothly bordered; it is also protruded and rounded. The pleural base may protrude; the margin towards the ventilated lung may be slightly constricted (Fig. 4.37).

In early infarctions, the central bronchial reflex is either weak or absent. This is, on the one hand, an expression of the well known bronchial constriction in cases of pulmonary embolism, and is caused on the other hand by compression of the surrounding accumulation of edemas and hematomas. A distinctive air bronchogram is not seen in any early lung infarction (Mathis et al 1993; Mathis and Dirschmid 1993).

Late Pulmonary Infarction, Tissue Necrosis

The *late pulmonary infarction* is more coarse and grainy in structure than the fresh infarction. It has sharp, serrated margins, is frequently triangular or wedge-shaped, more rarely rounded or quadrangular. In most cases, it is somewhat more echodense than the early infarction and has a pronounced central bronchial reflex which, on cross-section, is found in the center of the triangle and is a sign of segmental infestation. Small lung infarctions of up to 2 cm in size often have no bronchial reflex. They remain hypoechoic and homogeneous until their margins tend to become blurred (Figs. 4.38–4.40; Table 4.8).

Table 4.8. Sonomorphology of pulmonary infarctions

Early infarction	Late infarction
Homogeneous	Inhomogeneous/grained
Round > triangular	Triangular > round
Smooth margins	Serrated margins
Sparse internal echoes	Segmental bronchial reflex
Circulation stop	Vascular signs

In lesions less than 2 cm in size, these criteria apply to a very limited extent.

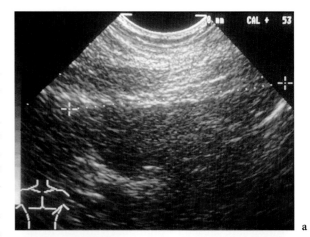

a

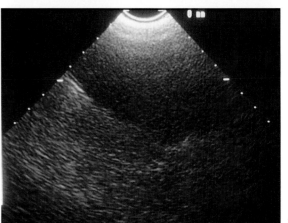

b

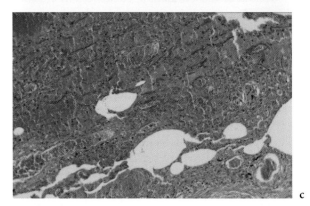

c

Fig. 4.37. **a** A fresh pulmonary infarction (+...+) 2 h after the embolism occurred in the anterobasal lung. Hypoechoic texture with initial echoes, rounded towards the hilum. The position, form, and early stage were confirmed by autopsy and histology. **b** The same early pulmonary infarction in a water bath: a largely homogeneous lesion. **c** Histology reveals that the alveolar spaces are congested with erythrocytes, but the structure of the lung is fully preserved

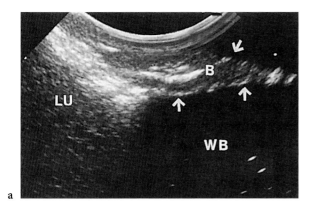

a

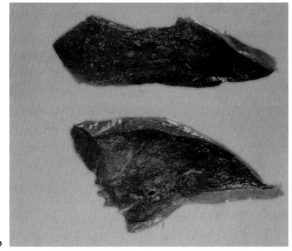

b

Fig. 4.38. a Old pulmonary infarction (*arrows*) in an autopsied lung in a water bath. *B*, bronchial reflex; *LU*, ventilated lung; *WB*, water bath. **b** Macropathology of the same pulmonary infarction which was also confirmed by histology

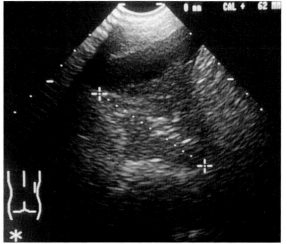

a

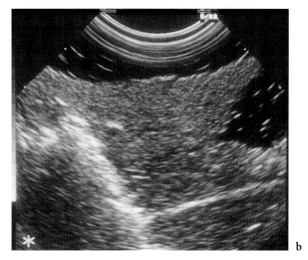

b

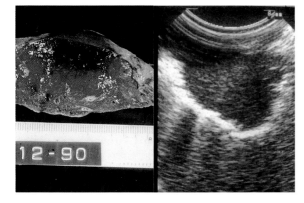

Fig. 4.39. Classical pulmonary infarction with tissue necrosis in the autopsied lung (*left*). Ultrasonographic image in a water bath (*right*)

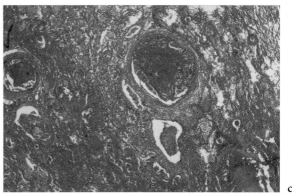

c

Fig. 4.40. a Old quadrangular pulmonary infarction (+...+) with a moderately dense and somewhat coarse echotexture. This form is also characteristic for the vascular supply. In the center, there is a broad bronchial reflex. **b** In the water bath, this pulmonary infarction is echogenic and coarse-grained. **c** Histology reveals congested thromboembolic vessels and tissue necrosis

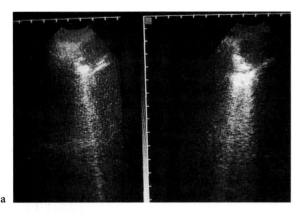
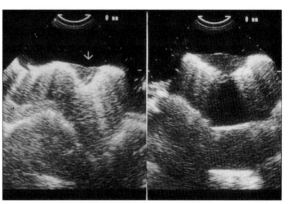

a   b

Fig. 4.41a, b. This patient was admitted to hospital for treatment of 3-layered thrombosis in the veins of the leg. After he was physically mobile he suffered a cardiovascular arrest. During reanimation, several signal embolisms were seen on ultrasonographic images obtained with a bedside unit. **b** In terms of position, form, and size the embolisms were confirmed on autopsy as well as in the water bath

Signal Embolisms

A massive pulmonary embolism is frequently accompanied by smaller embolic events, which then appear as *signal embolisms*. They are visualized as individual triangular or rounded small lesions (Fig. 4.41). Several such small defects lying adjacent to each other create the image of a lacerated margin between the nonventilated portion of the lung lying close to the pleura and the normally ventilated portion of the lung. Such small lesions may be an early sign of imminent pulmonary embolism or may even be present in conjunction with a massive central pulmonary embolism and thus confirm the diagnosis without the central embolus itself being demonstrated on chest sonography. This escapes demonstration because of intermediate air (Kroschel et al. 1991; Mathis 1992).

Vascular Signs

In some cases, a *vascular band* is seen on the B-mode image. The vascular band extends from the tip of the lesion towards the hilum. It corresponds to the congested thromboembolic branch of the pulmonary artery, which is also seen in CT examinations (vessel sign or vascular sign) (Ren et al. 1990) (Fig. 4.42, see also Fig. 4.46 f).

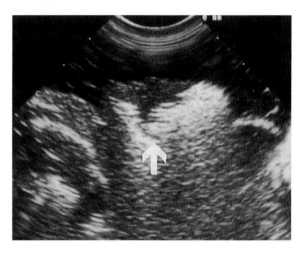

Fig. 4.42. Pulmonary infarction with "vascular signs" in a water bath. Histology showed that it was a recent pulmonary infarction. The supplying vessel was congested by thromboembolism

Pleural Effusion

In approximately half of all cases, the investigator finds small pleural effusions, either focally above the lesion or in the pleural sinuses. The effusion is largely anechoic and small compared to a lesion caused by infarction, which is an important criterion to distinguish this entity from compression atelectasis.

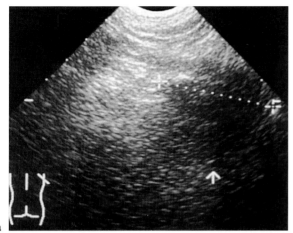

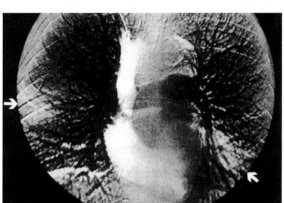

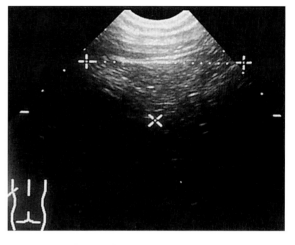

The pleural effusion may also lead to an apparent echo enhancement in the pulmonary infarction. Internal echoes in the effusion and fibrin strands are indicative of infarction pneumonia (Mathis et al. 1993) (Figs. 4.43–4.52).

Fig. 4.44. A hyperechoic triangular recent pulmonary infarction (5.5 × 3 cm) is very rare. The echo dense image may have been due to hemorrhagic congestion, as has also been observed in some hematomas. This finding was also verified on angiography

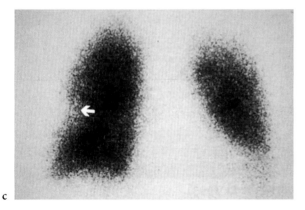

Fig. 4.43. a Somewhat blurred margins, hypoechoic, largely homogeneous recent pulmonary infarction in a lateral location on the right side. The pleural surface of the infarction is slightly protruded. **b** This (female) patient's angiogram of the pulmonary artery shows two interruptions of the vessel due to pulmonary embolism. **c** The lung scintigram of this patient only reveals a perfusion defect. The second pulmonary infarction was seen on sonography as well as angiography

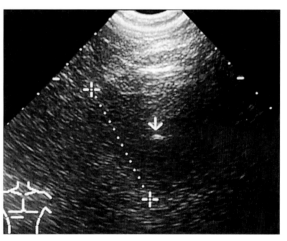

Fig. 4.45. The central bronchial reflex (*arrow*) is very small in recent pulmonary infarctions, if it is present at all. Notably, once the initial echo is omitted, the texture here is also hypoechoic and largely homogeneous

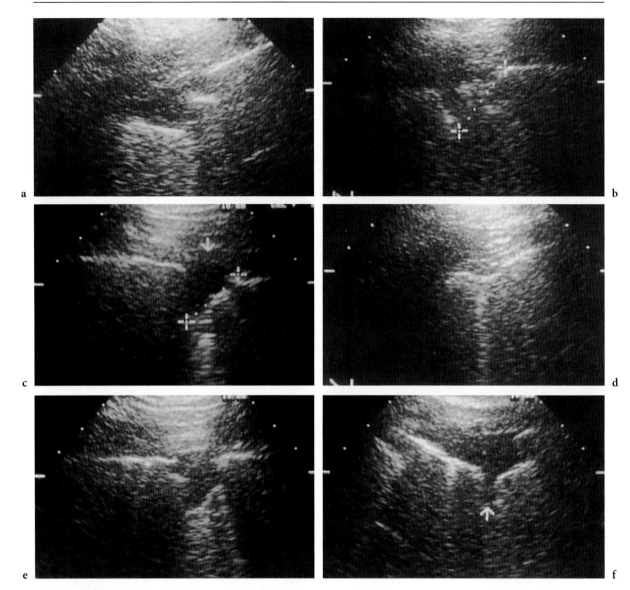

Fig. 4.46 a–f. This male patient had a three-layered leg vein thrombosis. After an episode of dyspnea, a sensation of pressure in the rib cage, and coughing, six pulmonary infarctions of between 2 and 3 cm in size (**a–f**) were seen on sonography – typical signal embolisms. They are largely wedge-shaped. In Fig. **c** (*arrow*) the pleural protrusion is clearly visible. Infarctions of this size escape detection by scintigraphy, especially those as in Fig. **d**. In this case scintigraphy showed two perfusion defects. The supplying vessel filled with thromboembolism is well depicted in Fig. **f** (*arrow*)

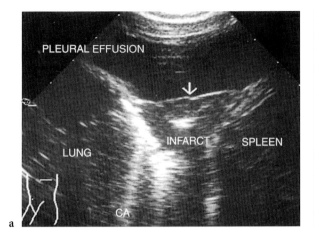 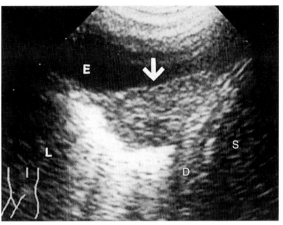

Fig. 4.47. a Five-day-old pulmonary infarction. Sharp margins, somewhat more echo dense and more coarsely structured than in the early stage, with a pronounced central bronchial reflex. *CA*, comet-tail artifact. **b** The same lesion in longitudinal section. The echogenicity is somewhat enhanced also by the pleural effusion (*E*). *L*, ventilated lung; *D*, diaphragm; *S*, spleen

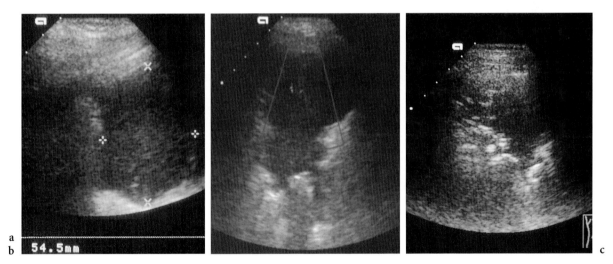

Fig. 4.48. a Five hours after the embolic event, a rounded homogeneous early infarction is seen. **b** After 5 days, the lesion is triangular. **c** After 12 days, a classical pulmonary infarction has developed. It is somewhat smaller than the original lesion, triangular in shape and has serrated margins

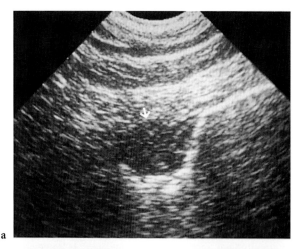

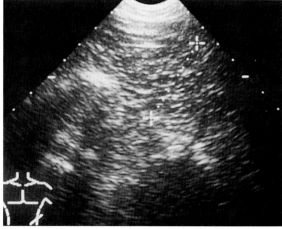

a

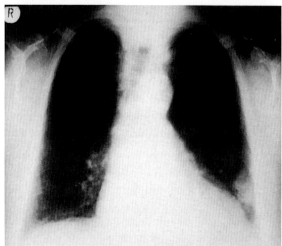

b

Fig. 4.50. Old pulmonary infarction 15 days after the incident. The area is partially reventilated, very coarsely structured, and has blurred margins. At this stage, a distinction between this condition and pneumonia (including infarction pneumonia) cannot be made on the basis of sonomorphology. This patient had no clinical symptoms of pneumonia

Fig. 4.49. a Older pulmonary infarction. Even without the presence of a pleural effusion, the protrusion of the pleural surface of the infarction is well depicted (*arrow*). **b** This infarction was seen on ultrasonography 4 days before it was visualized on the fluoroscopic chest radiograph

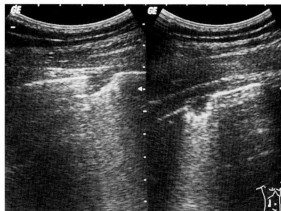

a

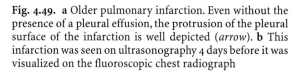

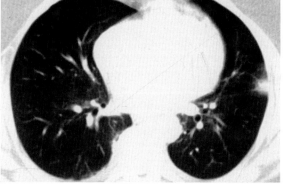

b

Fig. 4.51. A 25-year-old woman with sudden dyspnea and mild respiration-related chest pain. **a** Sonography reveals two small pulmonary infarctions. **b** On spiral CT, the central pulmonary embolism is confirmed and only one focus is seen in the periphery

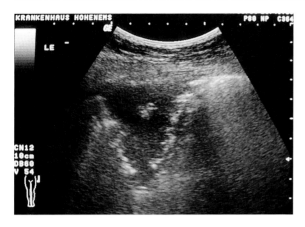

Fig. 4.52. Large classical pulmonary infarction with saw-tooth margins and a central bronchial reflex

Color-Coded Duplex Sonography in Pulmonary Embolism

Only in very few cases is the investigator able to visualize, on color-coded duplex sonography, a circulation stop caused by embolism (Fig. 4.53). This limitation has several reasons:

- When early reperfusion occurs, the lesion is revascularized early.
- Patients with dyspnea cannot hold their breath long enough, which causes several artifacts on color-coded duplex sonography.
- It is difficult to locate the supplying vessel at the right level.

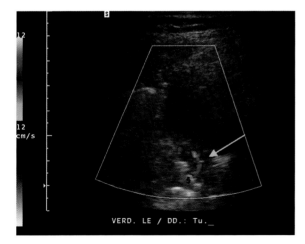

Fig. 4.53. Circulation stop at the tip of the wedge

Initial encouraging results achieved with color-coded duplex sonography in the differential diagnosis of peripheral lung consolidations have not been sufficiently evaluated and/or verified (Yuan et al. 1993; Gehmacher and Mathis 1994).

Healing Phase – Infarction Pneumonia

Several weeks after a pulmonary embolism, the sonomorphology of the pulmonary infarction is no longer characteristic. As reventilation progresses, the sonographic image resembles that of pneumonia (Fig. 4.50). Infarction pneumonias may develop in the vicinity of the infarction or even between multiple infarctions. Coughing up sequestrated infarctions creates infarction cavities, which may become subject to secondary infection and lead to a pulmonary abscess.

Therefore, the processes of repair of late infarctions offer very different conditions for ultrasonographic imaging. A sonomorphological distinction between this entity and other peripheral lung consolidations now becomes difficult. In cases that arrive for ultrasonographic investigation in the stage of infarction pneumonia, 1–2 weeks after the event, the lesion can be imaged by ultrasonography, but the sonomorphology offers very few criteria for differential diagnosis.

Sonomorphological Differential Diagnosis

Various criteria permit sonomorphological differential diagnosis between pneumonia and peripheral pulmonary lesions of other origin. *Pneumonias* have blurred margins on the sonogram, are inhomogeneously structured, have numerous lenticular internal echoes, air bronchograms, and in cases of poststenotic pneumonias even fluid bronchograms. In the early stage, pneumonia may be similar to the liver. However, in most cases, they are smaller than on chest radiographs, as air echoes tend to artificially obliterate the image in terms of depth. If pneumonias are larger than on radiographs, the magnification is nearly always due to effusion (see Sect. 4.1).

Carcinomas and metastases are rather rounded or polycyclic, grow in an invasive fashion, have crow's feet, tumor cones, and occasionally central necroses.

Compression atelectases are narrow, shaped like a pointed cap, concave on at least one side, and float

Table 4.9. Chest sonography in the diagnosis of pulmonary embolism

Author	Year	Patients (n)	Sensitivity (%)	Specificity (%)	PPV (%)	NPV (%)	Accuracy (%)	Reference methods
Mathis et al.	1990	33	96	60	93	75	91	Scintigraphy, angiography
Kroschet al.	1991	100	90	81	100	81	93	Scintigraphy
Mathis et al.	1993	58	98	66	91	89	90	Scintigraphy, angiography
Lechleitner et al.	1997	119	86	67	55	91	73	Scintigraphy, d-dimer testing
Mathis et al.	1999	117	94	87	92	91	91	Spiral CT
Reisig et al.	2000	69	80	92	95	72	84	Spiral CT
Lechleitner et al.	2000	55	81	84	97	84	82	MRI

PPV, positive predictive value; *NPV*, negative predictive value; *CT*, computed tomography; *MRI*, magnetic resonance imaging.

in the effusion, which is much larger than atelectasis (Mathis et al. 1993; Mathis 1997).
Color-coded duplex sonography is also suitable for differentiating between pneumonic and neoplastic lesions: pneumonias have an enhanced, regular central pattern of circulation, while carcinomas and metastases are nourished by atypical corkscrew-shaped vessels that flow from the margin.

Accuracy of Chest Sonography in the Diagnosis of Pulmonary Embolism

A total of 75% of hemorrhages and infarctions resulting from pulmonary embolism occur in the lower lobes of the lung and usually in a dorsal location at this site, i.e., in an area that is readily accessible to thorax sonography.
So far, seven prospective studies of 551 patients have dealt with the accuracy of chest sonography in the diagnosis of pulmonary embolism (Table 4.9). In all investigations concerning the diagnosis of pulmonary embolism, the problem is the virtual absence of a gold standard. Nevertheless, it is obvious that similar results have been achieved with different comparable methods. The overall sensitivity of chest sonography is 90% and the specificity 80%, which is sufficient documentation of the clinical value of the method.

Thorax Sonography in the Context of Other Imaging Procedures

Chest Radiograph

The chest radiograph, which is the basic imaging procedure in the diagnosis of lung disease, is known to be very unreliable in cases of pulmonary embolism. It serves the purpose of interpreting scintigraphic findings and may be a reason to perform a chest sonography. Chest radiographs are used to exclude other diseases and are, as a general rule, normal (Mathis et al. 1993).

Ventilation/Perfusion Scintigraphy

Since the largest study concerning the value of V/P scintigraphy was performed, the value of this method in the diagnosis of pulmonary embolism has been controversial. It was found that only a minority of patients (11%) in whom a pulmonary embolism was eventually proven by angiography had a V/P scintigraphy with a high diagnostic probability. Three quarters of patients needed further investigations to confirm or exclude a pulmonary embolism (PIOPED Investigators 1990). Nevertheless, scintigraphy is much more widely accepted and further studies in small groups of patients, some with altered diagnostic criteria, have shown better results. However, the basic method-based problem remains: small peripheral perfusion defects measuring up to 2 cm in size escape detection by scintigraphy. Whether these small signal embolisms are harmless or are predictors of a life-threatening pulmonary embolism is not yet established. A European-wide review mainly comprising German, British, and French studies showed that ventilation/perfusion scintigraphy on a 24-h basis is only available in 14.6% of the institutions (Köhn and Köhler 1989).

A comparison between scintigraphy and chest sonography revealed a high degree of concurrence between scintigraphy and ultrasonography for high-probability scans. However, on intermediate- and low-probability scans, typical embolic lesions were seen more clearly on sonography (Mathis et al. 1990; Kroschel et al. 1991; Lechleiner et al. 1997). On the other hand, a few large perfusion defects on scintigraphy had no correlate on sonography. This is in agreement with the unsatisfying results of the PIOPED study, in which only a small minority (sensitivity, 41%) of patients had pulmonary embolism scans of high probability while 33% of those with intermediate and 12% of those with low probability scans eventually had a pulmonary embolism. Eminent authors recommend refraining from using scintigraphy in such cases (Goodman and Lipchik 1996).

Spiral Computed Tomography

Spiral CT has revolutionized the diagnosis of pulmonary embolism. It is the first method to provide a means of almost entirely noninvasive and direct imaging of the embolus. In initial studies, spiral CT demonstrated a very high sensitivity (91%–100%) and specificity in the diagnosis of acute pulmonary embolism (Remy-Jardin et al. 1992; Teigen et al. 1993). According to recent investigators, however, the accuracy is markedly lower (Rathbun et al. 2000). Central pulmonary embolisms up to the level of segmental arteries are diagnosed or excluded with great certainty on spiral CT. In segmental arteries, however, spiral CT approaches its limits as a diagnostic procedure. One third of lung embolisms escape detection even by this method, especially those in the segmental region, particularly when indirect signs of peripheral consolidations are not additionally reported on (Goodman et al. 1996; Mathis et al. 1999). Their characteristic form is known from conventional CT (Ren et al. 1990). When indirect signs are taken into account, the sensitivity can be markedly increased (Fig. 4.51). Comparing transthoracic sonography with spiral CT, which is currently regarded as the noninvasive method of choice by several authors, transthoracic sonography has an accuracy of about 90%. Thromboembolism in vessels is evidenced by spiral CT in 67%. This figure coincides with recent data in the literature, in which one third of embolisms, namely those in the subsegmental region, are not detected by spiral CT (Oser et al. 1996). When subpleural consolidations seen on spiral CT are additionally evaluated, the sensitivity of spiral CT increases to 85%. In terms of shape and size, infarctions are visualized in a similar way as on CT. It was also found out that sonography and spiral CT complement each other, as chest sonography shows high sensitivity, especially in cases of small peripheral lesions.

Pulmonary Angiography

Angiography of the pulmonary artery is still considered the "gold standard" in the diagnosis of pulmonary embolism. Even the PIOPED study did not improve the acceptance of pulmonary artery angiography: patients with intermediate and low-probability scans are no longer subjected to angiographic investigation even in large centers. Furthermore, the invasive nature of the procedure prohibits wide application. Invasive procedures are an ethical problem since a noninvasive method like spiral CT (that was initially very promising in terms of accuracy) has become available. Investigators differ greatly in terms of their evaluation of peripheral vascular interruptions. The pulmonary infarction seen on sonography is 1–2 cm smaller than that on angiography (see Fig. 4.43), as the mantle zone of the infarction is sufficiently nourished by collateral vessels. Several small and angiographically verified defects that are indicative of a normal scintigram can be imaged by sonography.

The Sonographic Search for the Source of Embolism

In other anatomical locations, ultrasonography has become the method of choice for diagnosing thromboembolism. In a single investigation and with one imaging system, the experienced investigator is able to inspect several actual clinically or potentially involved regions of the body. He is able to study the source, pathway, and target of the embolic event.

Duplex Sonography of Leg Veins

Far more than half of all pulmonary embolisms originate from leg veins. In autopsies of 837 adults, the incidence of pelvic/leg vein thrombosis was 39%. Of these, 56% also had a pulmonary embolism (Feigl and Schwarz 1978). Among 105 patients with confirmed leg vein thrombosis, the prevalence of pulmonary embolism was 57%, while it was only 4.7% in patients without leg vein thrombosis. A closer look at the source of embolism reveals the following prevalence of pulmonary embolism: 46% in patients with calf thrombosis, 67% in the thigh, and 77% in pelvic vein thrombosis (Köhn and Scheibal 1978).

Duplex sonography with compression is a safe procedure to confirm the source of embolism from a deep vein thrombosis. In cases of suspected leg vein thrombosis, the median sensitivity is 95% (range, 38%–100%) and the median specificity, 97% (range, 81%–100%). Even in cases of the relatively frequent isolated lower leg thrombosis, the median sensitivity is 89% (range, 36%–96%) and the median specificity, 92% (range, 50%–98%) (Jäger et al. 1993). Visualization of the thrombus and the absence of flow are direct signs of leg vein

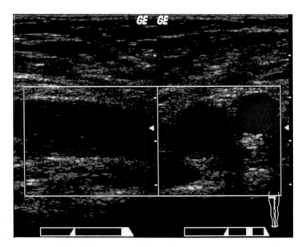

Fig. 4.54. Search for the source of embolism: Leg vein thrombosis in the femoral vein. The vein is larger than the artery, congested with echogenic material, and noncompressible. The margins reveal minimal flow

thrombosis (Fig. 4.54). Detection of the thrombus in the B mode is indirectly improved by the application of color Doppler. Several indirect signs improve accuracy. The thrombosed vein is not compressible or only partially compressible, which is indicative of an occluding or surrounded coagulation. However, signs of compressibility are only reliable when they are found in the inguinal or popliteal region. The vena cava and pelvic veins are not sufficiently compressible. In cases of calf thrombosis the compression is painful on palpation. The respiratory phase of venous flow is lost at a location distal to any hindrance of flow. In cases of acute thrombosis the vein is markedly dilated and valvular movements are absent. A careful comparison between the veins of one leg and those of the other is essential (Table 4.10; Eichlisberger 1995).

Table 4.10. Duplex sonography of deep vein thrombosis in the leg. (From Eichlisberger 1995)

	Method of detection
Direct signs	
Visible thrombus	B-mode image
No flow	PW-Doppler, color
Indirect signs	
Noncompressible vein	B-mode image
Flow signals not related to the respiratory phase	PW-Doppler, color
Flow signals not spread over the entire cross-section	Color
Larger diameter (acute TVT)	B-mode image
Collateral veins	B-mode image, color
Missing valvular movement	B-mode image
Not extensible using Valsalva's maneuver	B-mode image

Echocardiography

Since the introduction of transesophageal echo-cardiography, the *heart* has also been frequently studied as a *source of embolism*. In the right atrium, transthoracic echocardiography reveals sessile and floating thrombi (Fig. 4.55), occasionally even riding thrombi in the main central branches of pulmonary arteries (Kronik et al. 1989; Vuille et al. 1993). In cases of submassive and massive pulmonary embolism, the right heart reveals characteristic changes on echocardiography:

- Dilatation of the right atrium
- Dilatation of the right ventricle
- Paradoxical movement of the septum, flattening of the septum
- Tricuspid insufficiency > 2.5 m/s
- Increased pulmonary artery pressure > 39 mm Hg

A major advantage of sonographic investigation of embolism is its manifold applicability and its availability at the bedside, whether in the emergency department or on the intensive care unit.

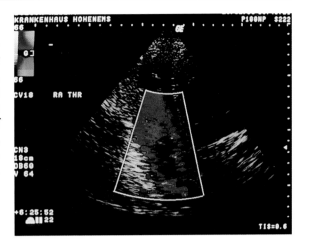

Fig. 4.55. Floating thrombus in the right heart. In the course of the recurring thromboembolic event, the floating thrombus has disappeared. Chest sonography showed small signal emboli

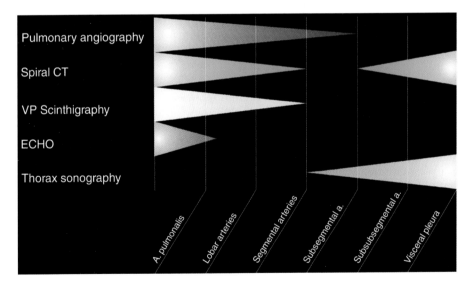

Fig. 4.56. Comparison of methods for diagnosing pulmonary embolism. *CT*, computed tomography; *VP*, ventilation/perfusion. (Modified according to Kroschel et al. 1991; Kroegel and Reißig 2000)

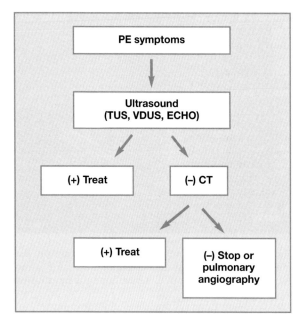

Fig. 4.57. Procedure in cases of clinically suspected pulmonary embolism (*PE*). In individual cases, ventilation/perfusion scintigraphy might provide additional information. *TUS*, transcutaneous ultrasonography; *VDUS*, vein duplex ultrasonography. (Modified according to Goodman 1996)

Summary

When a pulmonary embolism develops, transthoracic sonography usually reveals subpleural sound-permeable lesions. These are, on the one hand, embolism-related alveolar edemas that can be reperfused, and hemorrhages (early pulmonary infarctions). On the other hand, the lesions may be marked pulmonary infarctions that have a characteristic sonomorphological appearance: wedge-shaped, with a pleural base, with sharp margins and with a central bronchial reflex. The specificity of the method, however, is limited and *a normal chest sonography does not exclude pulmonary embolism* (Figs. 4.56 and 4.57).

References

Ducker EA, Rivitz SM, Shepard JAO et al. (1998) Acute pulmonary embolism: assessment of helical CT for diagnosis. Radiology 209:235–241

Eichlisberger R, Frauchinger B, Holtz D, Jäger KA (1995) Duplexsonographie bei Verdacht auf tiefe Venenthrombose und zur Abklärung der Varikose. In: Jäger KA,

Eichlisberger R (Hrsg) Sonokurs. Karger, Basel, S 137–147

Feigl W, Schwarz N (1978) Häufigkeit von Beinvenenthrombosen und Lungenembolien im Obduktionsgut. In: Ehringer H (ed) Aktuelle Probleme in der Angiologie 33. Huber, Bern: pp 27–37

Gehmacher O, Mathis G (1994) Farkodierte Duplexsonographie peripherer Lungenherde – ein diagnostischer Fortschritt? Bildgebung 61:S2:11

Goldhaber SZ, Visani L, De Rosa M (1999) Acute pulmonary embolism: clinical outcomes in the International Cooperative Pulmonary Embolism Registry. Lancet 353: 9162, 1386–1389

Goodman LR, Curtin JJ, Mewissen MW et al. (1995) Detection of pulmonary embolism in patients with unresolved clinical and scintigrafic diagnosis: helical CT versus angiography. AJR 164:1369–1374

Goodman LR, Lipchik RJ (1996) Diagnosis of pulmonary embolism: Time for a new approach. Radiology 199: 25–27

Hartung W (1984) Embolie und Infarkt. In: Remmele W (Hrsg) Pathologie 1. Springer, Berlin Heidelberg New York Tokyo, S 770–772

Heath D, Smith P (1988) Pulmonary embolic disease. In: Thurlbeck WM (ed) Pathology of the lung. Thieme, Stuttgart; pp 740–743

Jäger K, Eichlisberger R, Frauchinger B (1993) Stellenwert der bildgebenden Sonographie für die Diagnostik der Venenthrombose. Haemostaseologie 13:116–123

Joyner CR, Miller LD, Dudrick SJ, Eksin DJ (1966) Reflected ultrasound in the detection of pulmonary embolism. Trans Ass Am Phys 79:262–277

Köhn H, Köhler D (1989) Diagnostic modalities for detection of pulmonary embolism in clinical routine. A European survey. In: Proceedings VIII Congress of the European Society of Pneumology. Freiburg

Könn G, Schejbal E (1978) Morphologie und formale Genese der Lungenthromboembolie. Verh Dtsch Ges Inn Med 84:269–276

Kroegel C, Reißig A (2000) Transthorakale Sonographie. Thieme, Stuttgart, S 82

Kronik G and The European working group (1989) The European cooperative study on the clinical significance of right heart thrombi. Eur Heart J 10:1046–1059

Kroschel U, Seitz K, Reuß J, Rettenmaier (1991) Sonographische Darstellung von Lungenembolien. Ergebnisse einer prospektiven Studie. Ultraschall Med 12:263–268

Lammers RJ, Bloor CM (1988) Pulmonary hemorrhage and infarction. In: Dail DH, Hammar SP (eds) Pulmonary pathology. Springer, Berlin Heidelberg New York Tokyo, pp 678–679

Lechleitner P, Raneburger W, Gamper G, Riedl B, Benedikt E, Theurl A (1998) Lung sonographic findings in patients with suspected pulmonary embolism. Ultraschall Med 19:78–82

Lechleitner P, Raneburger W, Gamper G, Riedl B, Benedikt E, Theurl A (1998) Lung sonographic findings in patients with suspected pulmonary embolism. Ultraschall Med 19:78–82

Mathis G, Metzler J, Fußenegger D, Sutterlütti G (1990a) Zur Sonomorphologie des Lungeninfarktes. In: Gebhardt J, Hackelöer BJ, von Klingräff G, Seitz K (Hrsg) Ultraschalldiagnostik '89. Springer, Berlin Heidelberg New York Tokyo, S 388–391

Mathis G, Metzler J, Feurstein M, Fußenegger D, Sutterlütti G (1990b) Lungeninfarkte sind sonographisch zu entdecken. Ultraschall Med 11:281–283

Mathis G, Metzler J, Fußenegger D, Sutterlütti G, Feurstein M, Fritzsche H (1993) Sonographic observation of pulmonary infarction and early infarctions by pulmonary embolism. Eur Heart J 14:804–808

Mathis G, Dirschmid K (1993) Pulmonary infarction: sonographic appearance with pathologic correlation. Eur J Radiol 17:170–174

Mathis G (1997) Thoraxsonography – Part II: Peripheral pulmonary consolidation. Ultrasound Med Biol 23:1141–1153

Mathis G, Bitschnau R, Gehmacher O et al. (1999) Chest ultrasound in diagnosis of pulmonary embolism in comparison to helical CT. Ultraschall Med 20:54–59

Miller LD, Joyner CR, Dudrick SJ, Eksin DJ (1967) Clinical use of ultrasound in the early diagnosis of pulmonary embolism. Ann Surg 166:381–392

Morgenthaler TI, Ryu JH (1995) Clinical characteristics of fatal pulmonary embolism in a referral hospital. Mayo Clin Proc 70:417–424

Morpurgo M, Schmid C (1995) The spectrum of pulmonary embolism. Clinicopathologic correlations. Chest 107 (Suppl 1):18S–20S

Oser RF, Zuckermann DA, Guttierrez FR, Brink JA (1996) Anatomic distribution of pulmonary emboli at pulmonary angiography: implications for cross-sectional imaging. Radiology 199:31–35

PIOPED Investigators (1990) Value of the ventilation/perfusion scan in acute pulmonary embolism. JAMA 263:2753–2759

Rathbun SW, Raskob GE, Whitsett TL (2000) Sensitivity and specificity of helical computed tomography in the diagnosis of pulmonary embolism: a systematic review. Ann Intern Med 132:227–232

Reißig A, Kroegel C (2000) Prospektive Untersuchung zur Diagnostik der Lungenembolie mittels transthorakaler Sonographie. Ultraschall Med 21:1–37

Remy-Jardin M, Remy J, Wattinne L, Giraud F (1992) Central pulmonary thromboembolism: Diagnosis with spiral volumetric CT with a single-breath-hold technique – comparison with pulmonary angiography. Radiology 185:381–387

Ren H, Kuhlman JE, Hruban RH, Fishman EK, Wheeler PS, Hutchins GM (1990) CT of infation-fixed lungs: wedge-shaped density and vasular sign in the diagnosis of infarction. J Comput Assist Tomogr 14:82–86

Teigen CL, Maus TP, Sheedy PF, Johnson CM, Stanson AW, Welch TJ (1993) Pulmonary embolism: diagnosis with electron-beam CT. Radiology 188:839–845

Vuille C, Urban P, Jolliet P, Louis M (1993) Thrombosis of the right auricle in pulmonary embolism: value of echocardiography and indications for thrombolysis. Schweiz Med Wochenschr 123:1945–1950

Yuan A, Yang PC, Chang CB (1993) Pulmonary infarction: use of color doppler sonography for diagnosis and assessment of reperfusion of the lung. AJR 160:419–420

4.4
Mechanical Lung Consolidations: Atelectasis

C. Görg

Definition

Atelectasis is defined as the absence of ventilation in portions of the lung or the entire lung. Such lack of ventilation may be permanent or transient, complete or partial (dystelectasis), congenital or acquired (Fig. 4.58).

Pathomorphology

Depending on the origin, a distinction is made between compression atelectasis and resorption atelectasis (obstructive atelectasis). Compression atelectasis may be anticipated when an accumulation of fluid causes intrapleural pressure to increase to a level higher than that of external air. This may be expected with an effusion of more than 2 l (Grundmann 1986).

Resorption atelectasis occurs when a bronchus is displaced in terms of its region of vascular supply, as a result of external compression or endobronchial obliteration.

In cases of resorption or obstructive atelectasis, a distinction is made between the central and peripheral form. Central obstruction is usually caused by endobronchial processes (e.g., bronchial carcinoma or foreign body) or extrabronchial alterations (e.g., enlarged lymph nodes), whereas peripheral bronchial obstructions are marked by inflammatory mucous plugs with displacement of small bronchial branches. Displacement of the lumen of the middle lobe by mucus or pus, scarred kinking of the bronchus, external lymph node compression, or tumor leads to the middle lobe syndrome.

Atelectasis impairs circulation in parenchyma, causing under-saturation of arteries due to reduced gas exchange in perfused, but not ventilated, atelectatic lung parenchyma.

In terms of pathological anatomy, the early phase of obstructive atelectasis is marked by fluid with a high protein content in intraalveolar spaces. The next stage is characterized by the migration of macrophages and lymphocytic infiltration. In cases of compression or even obstructive atelectasis

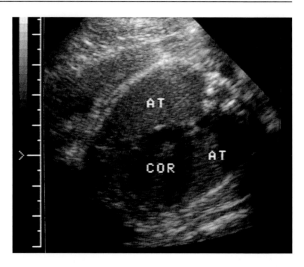

Fig. 4.58. Ultrasound through the thorax of a fetus at 32 weeks of gestation. Both lungs are homogeneous and hypoechoic – complete atelectasis (*AT*). *COR*, heart

of longer duration, there is a shrinking of parenchyma with fibrous induration of lung tissue.

Additional attendant phenomena or complications include retention of secretion in the presence of bronchial obstruction; bronchiectasis is seen in 40% of cases (Burke and Faser 1988; Yang et al 1990; Liaw et al 1994). In rare cases, the patient develops bacterial superinfection and microscopic or gross abscesses; necrotic or hemorrhagic foci in atelectatic tissue may also be found.

Sonomorphology

Lung atelectases are characterized by partial or complete absence of ventilation. Therefore, in principle, they can be imaged by sonography. Furthermore, the echo transparency of the lung permits the sonographer to evaluate the parenchyma. Especially in the presence of obstructive atelectasis, atelectatic lung tissue serves as "an acoustic window" for the investigation of central structures that possibly underlie the atelectasis.

Compression Atelectasis

The most common form is accompanied by the formation of pleural effusion. Depending on the extent of intrapleural fluid, the patient may develop homogeneous, hypoechoic transformations shaped like a wedge or a pointed cap (Fig. 4.59 a–c).

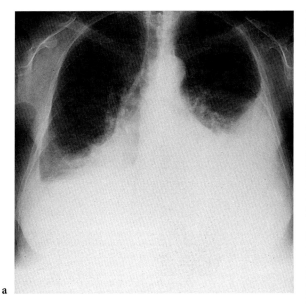

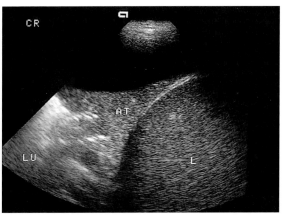

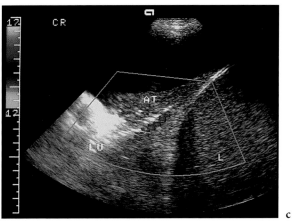

Fig. 4.59. a Chest radiograph of a 60-year-old man with global congestive heart failure and bilateral pleural effusions. **b** On ultrasonography, the right-lateral intercostal ultrasound beam transmission reveals a pleural effusion with a wedge-shaped hypoechoic transformation of portions of the lower lobe of the lung, corresponding to atelectasis (*AT*). The demarcation to ventilated lung tissue (*LU*) is blurred. An extensive air bronchogram is present (*L*, liver). **c** On color Doppler sonography, a flow signal is observed along the aerated bronchial branch

The margin to the adjacent aerated lung tissue is blurred. Usually, the atelectatic lung is surrounded by fluid, but also may be partly adherent to the pleura. The following features assist in the establishment of the diagnosis by sonography:

- Partial reventilation during inspiration (Fig. 4.60)
- Partial reventilation after puncture of effusion (Fig. 4.61)

During inspiration, sonography reveals an increasing quantity of air in atelectatic regions and the formation of a so-called air bronchogram. However, in the presence of exudative effusion, fibrin strands, septa, and echogenic pleural effusion, one frequently encounters impaired reventilation during inspiration, as a result of reduced elasticity of the lung. This condition has been described as a "trapped" lung (Lan et al. 1997).

Concomitant inflammatory invasion of parenchyma in atelectatic tissue is a further imitation. It leads to congestive pneumonia and restricts inspi-

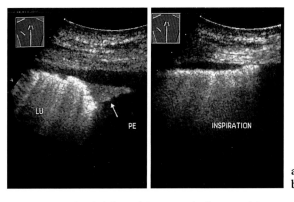

Fig. 4.60. a The left-lateral intercostal ultrasound beam transmission shows a pointed cap-like, smoothly margined, hypoechoic transformation at the tip of the lower lobe of the left lung (*LU*; *arrow*) in the presence of a pleural effusion (*PE*). **b** Deep inspiration results in reventilation of lung tissue as in compression atelectasis

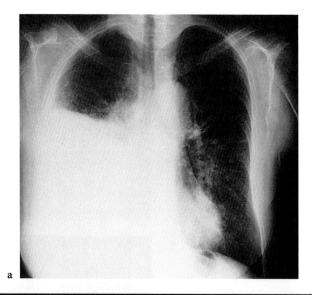

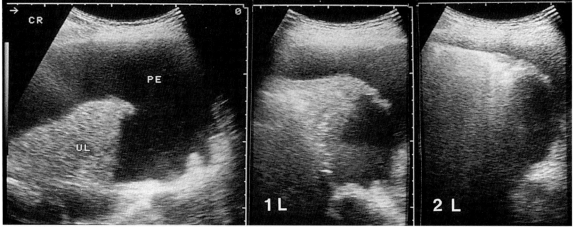

Fig. 4.61a, b. A 66-year-old man with alveolar cell carcinoma. **a** On chest radiograph, homogeneous opacity of the caudal portion of the right hemithorax is observed. **b** On ultrasonography, the right-lateral intercostal ultrasound beam transmission shows a marked pleural effusion (*PE*) with atelectasis of the lower lobe (*UL*). After puncture of the effusion (*central image 1 L*; *right image, 2 L*), ventilation is gradually restored, as in the presence of compression atelectasis

ratory ventilation. Based on sonomorphology alone, this condition cannot be distinguished from pneumonia (Fig. 4.62; Table 4.11).

In cases of compression atelectasis, lung tissue is partially re-ventilated after drainage of a perfusion. This is also dependent on the elasticity of the lung. Of course, ventilation of the parenchyma after puncture of an effusion does not rule out the possibility of an additional central space-occupying mass.

Table 4.11. Possible sonographic findings in the presence of compression atelectasis

---

B-mode sonography
- Moderate to marked pleural effusion
- Triangular, hypoechoic, pointed cap-like transformation of lung parenchyma
- Blurred margins to ventilated lung parenchyma
- Partial reventilation during inspiration (air bronchogram)
- Partial reventilation after puncture of effusion

Color Doppler sonography
- On intra-individual comparison with the liver, one finds enhanced flow phenomena

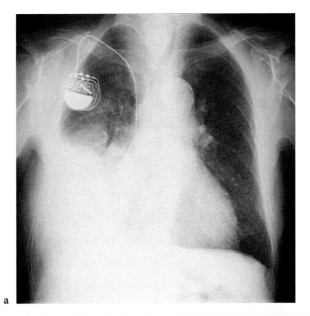

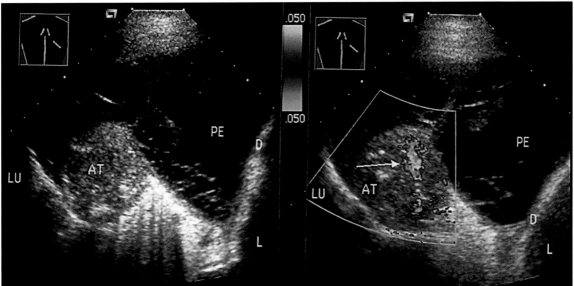

Fig. 4.62 a, b. A 75-year-old man with myocardial insufficiency. **a** Chest radiograph showed an opacity in the caudal portion of the right lung. **b** On ultrasonography (*left image*) the right-dorsal ultrasound beam transmission reveals a marked, partially septated pleural effusion (*PE*) and a circular hypoechoic consolidation in parts of the lung (*AT*). Color Doppler sonography (*right image*) shows marked flow signals. The marked pleural effusion and the absence of reventilation during inspiration raise suspicion of a fixed compression atelectasis. In principle, additional congestive pneumonia cannot be excluded on the basis of this image (*L*, liver; *LU*, lung; *D*, diaphragm)

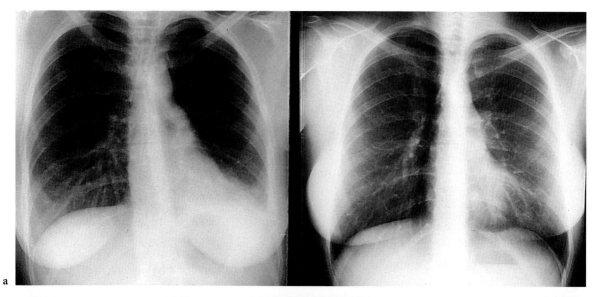

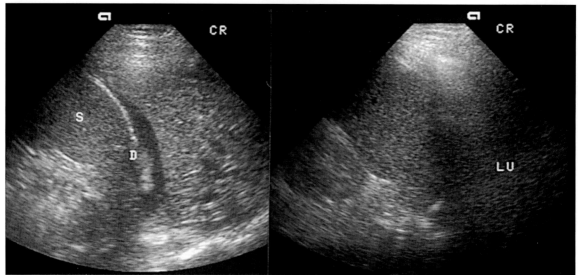

Fig. 4.63 a, b. A 20-year-old woman with fever and dyspnea. **a** Chest radiographs, show signs of atelectasis in the lower lobe on the left side (*left image*), which resolved spontaneously after 2 days (*right image*). **b** On ultrasonography, the left-lateral intercostal ultrasound beam transmission shows a homogeneous lung consolidation with a mild pleural effusion, as in the presence of obstructive atelectasis (*left image*). After 48 h, the lung is re-ventilated (*right image*). This is most likely due to displacement of a bronchus caused by an inflammatory mucous plug. *S*, spleen; *LU*, lung; *D*, diaphragm

Obstructive Atelectasis

The sonographic image of obstructive atelectasis is marked by a largely homogeneous, hypoechoic presentation of lung tissue in terms of hepatization (Figs. 4.63, 4.64). Effusion is absent or very mild. In cases of lobar atelectasis, the margin to ventilated lung tissue is rather distinct (Fig. 4.65).

Depending on the duration of atelectasis, intraparenchymatous structures may also be seen.

- Hypoechoic vascular lines and echogenic reflexes (Figs. 4.66, 4.67)
- Anechoic, hypoechoic, or echogenic focal lesions (Figs. 4.68, 4.69)

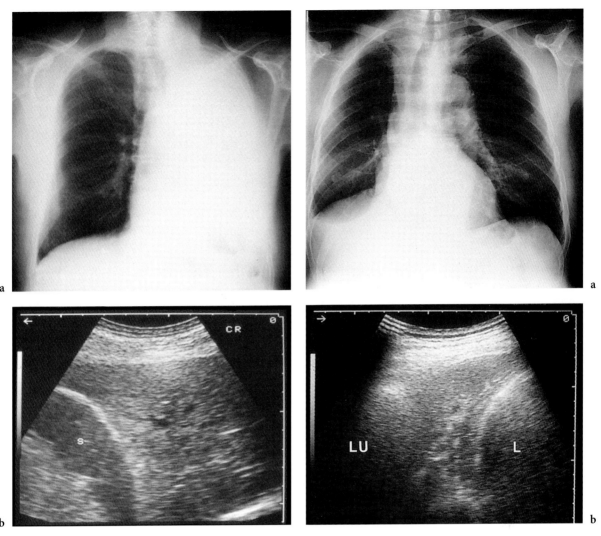

Fig. 4.64a, b. A 68-year-old man with bronchial carcinoma. **a** On chest radiograph, homogeneous opacity of the left-sided hemithorax can be observed. **b** On ultrasonography, the left-lateral intercostal ultrasound beam transmission shows a completely hypoechoic transformation of the left lung without effusion (so-called hepatization) in the presence of obstructive atelectasis. *S*, spleen

Fig. 4.66a, b. An 84-year-old man with bronchial carcinoma. **a** Chest radiograph shows predominantly right-sided lower lobe atelectasis. **b** On ultrasonography, the right-lateral intercostal ultrasound beam transmission shows a hypoechoic, poorly demarcated transformation with accentuated, hyperechoic reflexes in atelectatic lung tissue. *LU*, lung; *L*, liver

Fig. 4.65 see p. 78

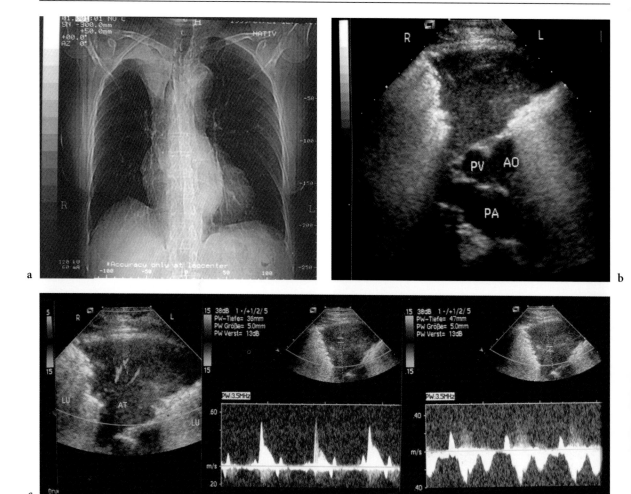

Fig. 4.65 a–c. A 74-year-old woman with dyspnea. **a** Chest radiograph shows signs of atelectasis of the upper lobe on the right side. **b** On ultrasonography, the right-ventral intercostal ultrasound beam transmission shows a smoothly margined, wedge-shaped transformation of the lung, as in the presence of atelectasis. Central vessels are imaged; a tumor core cannot be detected. *AO*, aorta; *PV*, pulmonary vein; *PA*, pulmonary artery. **c** Color Doppler sonography clearly shows arterial and venous flow profiles. Characteristic flow profiles of the pulmonary artery (*middle*) and pulmonary vein (*right*) are imaged

Fig. 4.66 see p. 77

Atelectasis of long duration is accompanied by sonographic reflexes in the lung parenchyma. The reflexes are caused by dilated bronchi, as a result of secretory congestion (so-called fluid bronchogram) (Fig. 4.70). Vessels along the bronchi are seen as branches of the pulmonary artery and pulmonary vein on color Doppler sonography (see Fig. 4.65; Table 4.12).

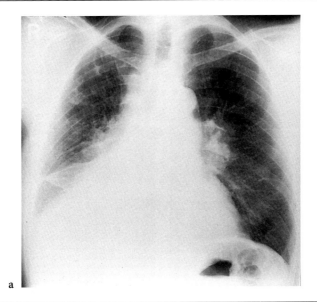

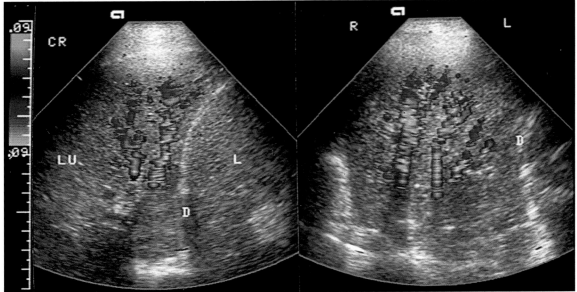

Fig. 4.67 a, b. A 58-year-old man with bronchial carcinoma. **a** Chest radiograph shows signs of right-sided lower lobe atelectasis. **b** On ultrasonography, the right-lateral intercostal ultrasound beam transmission reveals a hypo-echoic transformation of the lower lobe of the lung. Color Doppler sonography shows enhanced flow signals compared to the liver, which is typical evidence of atelectasis. *Lu*, lung; *D*, diaphragm; *L*, liver

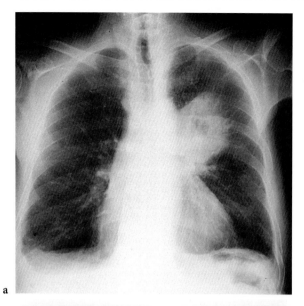

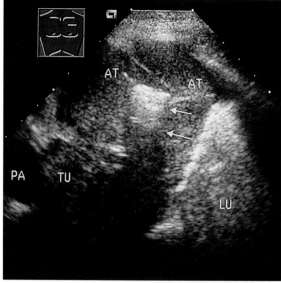

a   b

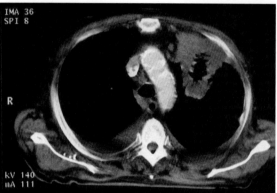

c

Fig. 4.68a–c. A 68-year-old man with bronchial carcinoma. **a** Chest radiograph shows a space-occupying mass in the left hilum and signs of formation of a central cavity. **b** On ultrasonography, the left-ventral intercostal ultrasound beam transmission shows upper lobe atelectasis (*AT*) and a tumor (*TU*) in the hilum, which can be distinguished from the atelectasis. In the central portion of atelectatic lung tissue, there is an aerated cavity (*arrows*) that is most likely representative of inflammatory retention. *LU*, lung; *PA*, pulmonary artery. **c** Computed tomography demonstrates atelectasis of the upper lobe with an aerated retention

Table 4.12. Possible sonographic findings in the presence of obstructive atelectasis

B-mode sonography	Color Doppler sonography
Mild or no pleural effusion	On intra-individual comparison with the liver, one finds enhanced flow phenomena
Homogeneous hypoechoic transformation of lung parenchyma	Triphasic spectrum of the arterial flow curve of pulmonary arteries (type: extremity arteries)
In some cases, hyperechoic reflexes may be found (fluid bronchogram)	
Occasionally, one may find foci within parenchyma	
Liquefaction of parenchyma	
Microabscesses or gross abscesses	
Metastases	
A central space-occupying mass may be visualized	
Absence of reventilation during inspiration	

Color Doppler Sonography

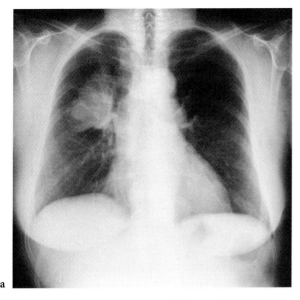

a

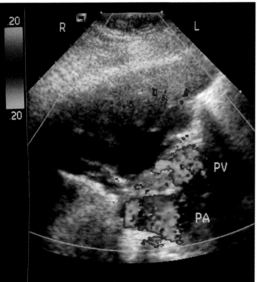

b

Fig. 4.69 a, b. The condition of a 63-year-old woman with a malignant lymphoma in the hilum after polychemotherapy and candidal pneumonia. **a** Chest radiograph shows a space-occupying mass in the central portion, in the right hilum. **b** On ultrasonography, The right-ventral intercostal ultrasound beam transmission shows partial atelectasis in the upper lobe. There is no tumor formation in the hilum. In the central portion of atelectatic lung tissue, there is an anechoic pseudocyst. On sonographic controls it has been constant for more than 12 months. *PV*, pulmonary vein; *PA*, pulmonary artery

On the sonogram, atelectatic lung tissue is marked by accentuated flow phenomena compared to the liver (Görg et al. 1996) (Fig. 4.67). Color Doppler sonography is limited by motion artifacts due to respiration and a possibly paracardiac position. Analysis of the venous Doppler flow curve will reveal the characteristic triphasic course of pulmonary veins.

Visualization of the arterial flow curve will show a triphasic spectrum as in the presence of high peripheral resistance (type: arteries of the extremities) with a steep increase in the systolic rate, a rapid fall in late systole, short diastolic backflow and late diastolic forward flow. Measurement of resistance will show high resistance (>0.80) and pulsatility (>250) indices (Yuan et al. 1994) (see Fig. 4.65).

Quite often, the investigator finds *focal lesions* in the lung parenchyma. As a result of dilated bronchi (due to congestion of secretion), one occasionally finds small anechoic, hypoechoic, or even echogenic foci within the parenchyma. Given corresponding clinical features, the foci are caused by microabscesses. Occasionally, the abscesses contain air echoes (Yang et al. 1992) (Fig. 4.68). Atelectasis caused by tumor often leads to intraparenchymatous liquefaction, which is seen on ultrasonography as large hypoechoic circular foci with characteristic motion echoes in "real-time" investigation. This is primarily due to necrosis or tumor-related retention of secretion. Abscesses cannot be entirely excluded on the basis of sonomorphology alone. Here, the clinical findings will be one of the main determinants of the diagnosis. However, ultrasound-guided puncture will allow the investigator to confirm the diagnosis and to obtain material for bacteriological investigation (Liaw et al. 1994) (see Chap. 7).

Occasionally, echogenic circular foci by way of metastases may be found in atelectatic lung tissue. They show intralesional flow signals on color Doppler sonography (see Chap. 7).

Essentially, in the presence of lobar or pulmonary atelectasis, central portions can be imaged through atelectatic lung tissue by sonography. The main purpose here is to demonstrate the central tumor if there is one. Based on sonographic structural features, a definite distinction between atelectatic lung tissue and tumor tissue can be made in less

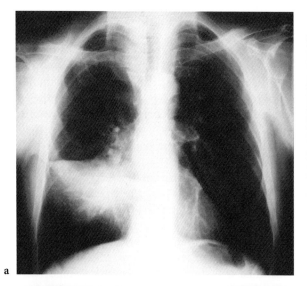

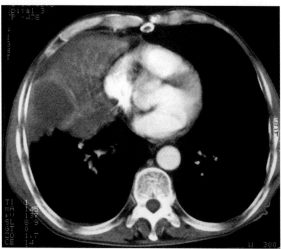

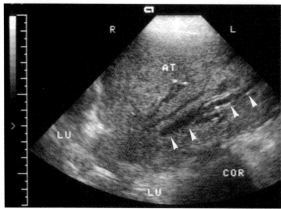

Fig. 4.70 a–c. A 68-year-old man with bronchial carcinoma. **a** Chest radiograph shows signs of middle lobe atelectasis. **b** On ultrasonography, the right-ventral intercostal ultrasound beam transmission shows middle lobe atelectasis and markedly dilated bronchi – a so-called fluid bronchogram ("sticks"). The central tumor is not clearly demarcated. *AT*, atelectasis; *LU*, lung; *COR*, heart. **c** Computed tomography demonstrated middle lobe atelectasis

than 50% of cases (Görg et al. 1996) (Figs. 4.71, 4.72). Additional color Doppler sonography may be helpful in this setting (Yuan et al. 1994), as tumor tissue is characterized by poor visualization of flow signals (Fig. 4.73). Measurement of resistance in arterial flow signals located within the tumor shows high diastolic flow and a correspondingly low resistance (RI < 0.8) and pulsatility index (PI < 2.50) (Yuan et al. 1994).

In a few cases, one finds central tumor spread into large vessels such as the aorta, the pulmonary artery and the pulmonary vein (Figs. 4.74, 4.75). The importance of visualizing the central tumor lies in the fact that the tumor can be punctured through atelectatic lung tissue under ultrasound guidance, with practically no risk of complications (Yang et al. 1990) (Fig. 4.76).

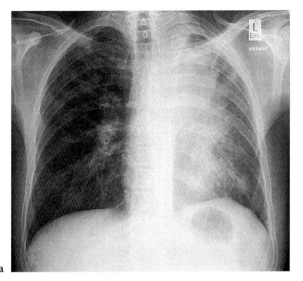

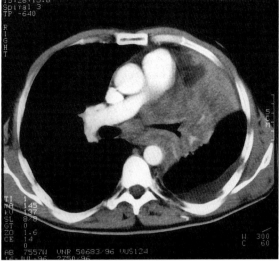

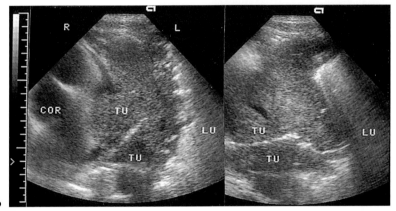

Fig. 4.71a–c. A 44-year-old man with bronchial carcinoma. **a** Chest radiograph shows signs of left-sided upper lobe atelectasis and dysatelectasis in the lower lobe. **b** On ultrasonography, the left-ventral intercostal ultrasound beam transmission shows atelectasis of the upper lobe. The central tumor formation (*TU*) is rather poorly differentiated from the atelectasis. The highly constricted bronchus is seen as an aerated band with abundant reflexes. *LU*, lung; *COR*, heart. **c** Computed tomography shows upper lobe atelectasis and the central tumor

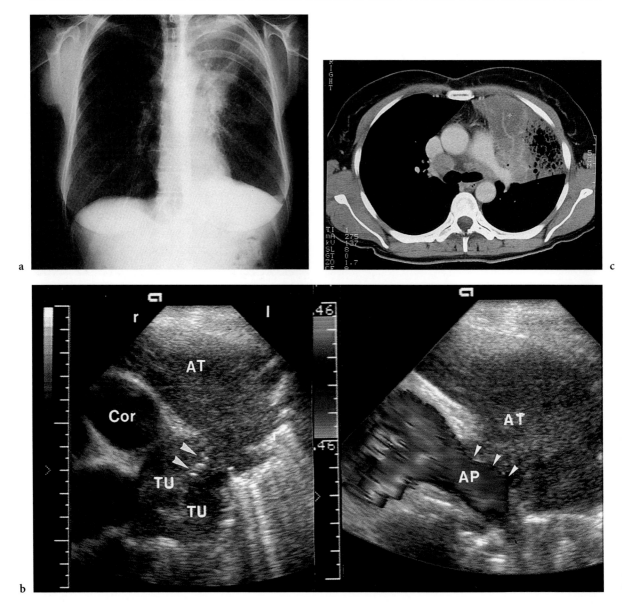

Fig. 4.72 a–c. A 48-year-old man with bronchial carcinoma. **a** Chest radiograph shows signs of atelectasis of the upper lobe on the left side. **b** On ultrasonography, the left-ventral intercostal ultrasound beam transmission shows upper lobe atelectasis (*AT*) and a central tumor (*TU*) that can be demarcated from it. On color Doppler sonography, the tumor is immediately adjacent to the pulmonary artery (*AP*) ("sticks"); *COR*, heart. **c** Computed tomography shows upper lobe atelectasis and the tumor entirely surrounding the pulmonary artery

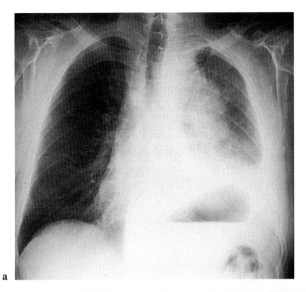

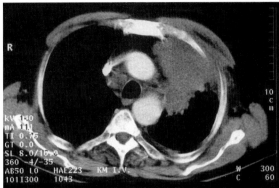

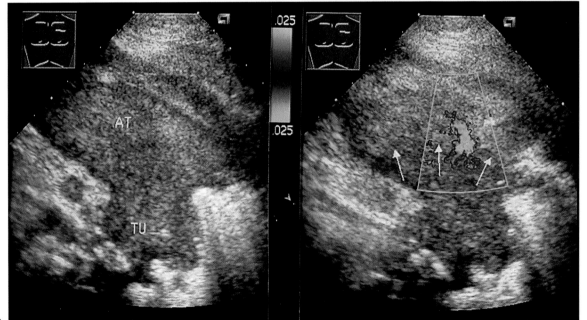

Fig. 4.73 a–c. A 70-year-old man with bronchial carcinoma. **a** Chest radiograph shows large tumor in the upper field on the left side. **b** On ultrasonography, hypoechoic tumor (*TU*) formation in the right upper lobe is seen, not clearly delineated from atelectatic lung tissue (*AT*). On color Doppler sonography, one finds strong evidence of flow signals in the peripheral portions (*arrows*), possibly a sign of atelectatic lung tissue. No flow signals are seen in the central portion of the tumor. **c** Computed tomography enables visualization of the tumor in the left hilum, as well as additional infiltration of the chest wall

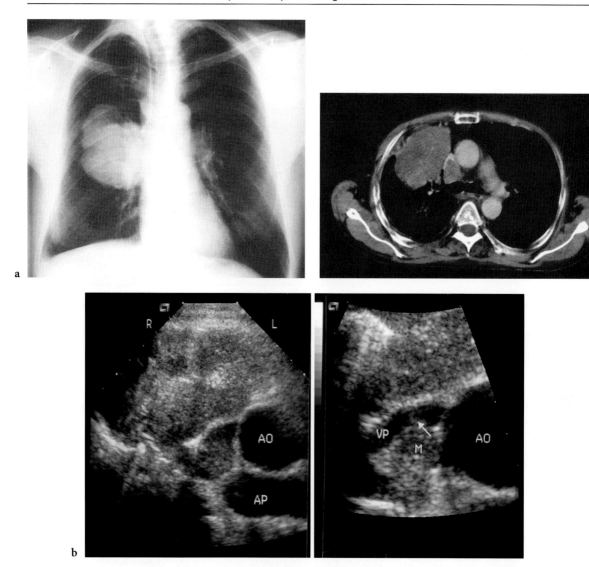

Fig. 4.74a–c. A 49-year-old man with bronchial carcinoma. **a** Chest radiograph shows central space-occupying mass in the right hilum. **b** On ultrasonography, the right-central intercostal ultrasound beam transmission shows a hypoechoic transformation. In terms of echomorphology, atelectatic lung tissue cannot be demarcated from the central tumor. In the aortopulmonary window one finds enlarged lymph nodes. Infiltration of the aorta (*AO*) cannot be excluded. *AP*, pulmonary artery; *VP*, pulmonary vein; *M*, lymph node metastasis. **c** Computed tomography demonstrates the tumor formation; it is touching the aorta

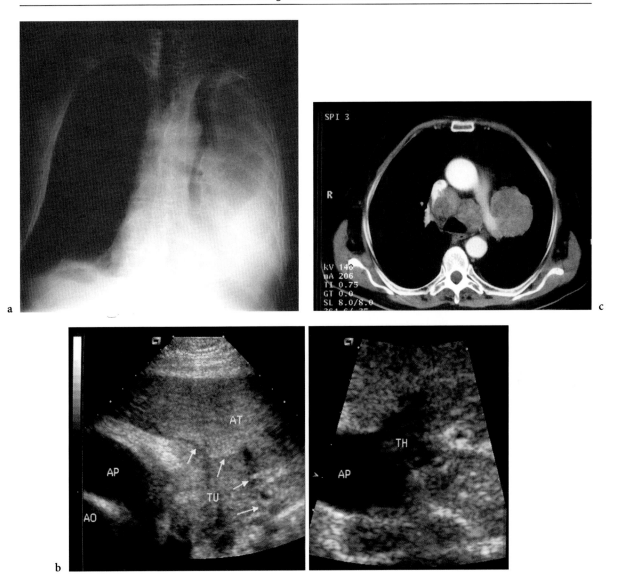

Fig. 4.75 a–c. A 77-year-old man with bronchial carcinoma. **a** Chest radiograph shows largely homogeneous opacity of the left hemithorax. **b** On ultrasonography, the left-ventral intercostal ultrasound beam transmission reveals a central tumor (*TU*) and atelectasis (*AT*). *Arrows* indicate the tumor margins where the atelectasis begins. Thrombotic material (*TH*) is found in the pulmonary artery (*AP*) (tumor thrombosis is suspected). **c** Computed tomography shows tumor development and contact with the aorta (*AO*)

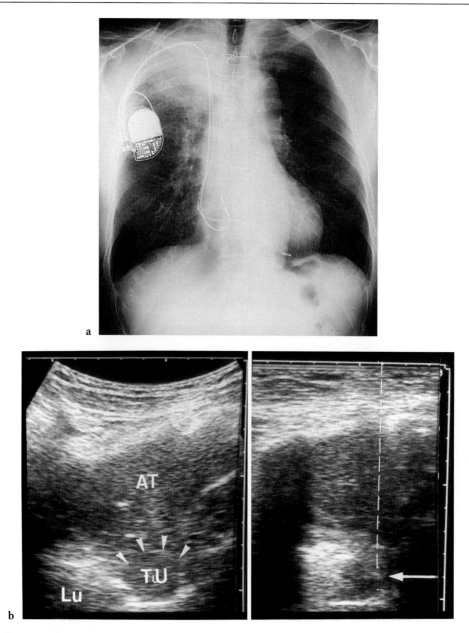

Fig. 4.76 a, b. A 67-year-old man with bronchial carcinoma. **a** Chest radiograph shows opacity in the upper lung
field on the right side. **b** On ultrasonography, the right-
ventral intercostal ultrasound beam transmission shows a
small central tumor (*TU*) with atelectasis (*AT*). Bronchoscopy did not reveal the tumor. Under ultrasound guidance, the tumor was punctured through atelectatic lung
tissue; a 16-gauge punch biopsy was performed. The *arrows*
show the reflex at the needle tip. Adenocarcinoma was
diagnosed. *LU*, lung

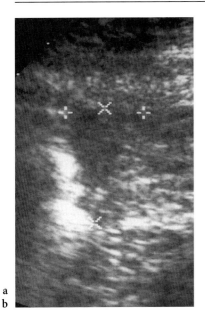
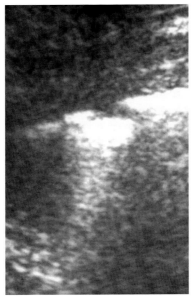
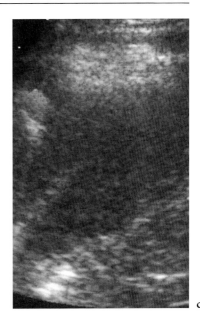

a
b
c

Fig. 4.77 a–c. Focal lung contusions following multiple rib fractures. Chest X-ray showed discrete areas of dystelectasia. The alterations seen on ultrasound are considerably more extensive: vague, poorly delimited, echo-poor subpleural areas

Lung Contusion

In cases of chest trauma, especially serial rib fractures, pulmonary contusions are seen better on sonography than on radiographs. Alveolar edema and alveolar hemorrhage caused by trauma are visualized as moderately hypoechoic blurred lesions with indistinct margins (Fig. 4.77). These are more pronounced in the presence of concomitant minimal pleural effusions, but are also imaged on sonography in the absence of pleural effusion. In the event of any clinically relevant chest trauma, both radiographs and sonograms should be obtained (see also Chap. 2).

Summary

In compression atelectasis, depending on the extent of intrapleural fluid, there usually is a homogeneous, hypoechoic transformation most commonly in the lower lobe, shaped like a pointed cap or a wedge. Its border with the adjacent aerated lung tissue is blurred. The sonographic image of an obstructive atelectasis is marked by a largely homogeneous hypoechoic visualization of lung tissue by way of hepatization. Effusion is mild or nonexistent. In lobar atelectasis, the border with the aerated lung tissue is relatively sharp. Intraparenchymal structures are seen as hypoechoic vascular lines, echogenic bronchial reflex bands or foci.

References

Burke M, Fraser R (1988) Obstructive pneumonitis: A pathologic and pathogenetic reappraisal. Radiology 166: 699–704

Görg C, Weide R, Walters E, Schwerk WB (1996) Sonographische Befunde bei ausgedehnten Lungenatelektasen. Ultraschall Klin Prax 11:14–19

Grundmann E (Hrsg) (1986) Spezielle Pathologie. 7. Aufl. Urban & Schwarzenberg, München

Lan RS, Lo KS, Chuang ML, Yang CT, Tsao TC, Lee CM (1997) Elastance of the pleural space: A predictor for the outcome of pleurodesis in patients with malignant pleural effusion. Ann Intern Med 126:768–774

Liaw YS, Yang PC, Wu ZG et al. (1994) The Bacteriology of Obstructive Pneumonitis. Am J Respir Crit Care Med 149:1648–1653

Yang PC, Luh KT, Chang DB, Yu CJ, Kuo SM, Wu HD (1992) Ultrasonographic evaluation of pulmonary consolidation. Am Rev Respir Dis 146:757–762

Yang PC, Luh KT, Wu DH, Chang DB, Lee NL, Kuo SM, Yang SP (1990) Lung tumors associated with obstructive pneumonitis: US studies. Radiology 174:717–720

Yuan A, Chang DB, Yu CJ, Kuo SH, Luh KT, Yang PC (1994) Color Doppler sonography of benign and malignant pulmonary masses. AJR 163:545–549

4.5
Congenital Pulmonary Sequestration

G. Mathis

The very rare pulmonary sequestration underlines the value and importance of thorax sonography in neonatology and pediatrics. The neonate with this condition suffers from dyspnea and has a non-specific systolic murmur. On chest radiograph, one may find a tumor-like shadow. On sonography, the echo texture of the pulmonary sequestration is similar to that of the liver, with wide arteries and veins (Gudinchet and Anderegg 1989). The supplying artery with the characteristic flow pattern can be identified on color-coded duplex sonography and the diagnosis is thus confirmed (Yuan et al. 1992). CT does not provide more information. If the lesion is imaged well on sonography, the infant can be spared the stress of angiography (Fig. 4.78).

References

Gudinchet F, Anderegg A (1989) Echography of pulmonary sequestration. Europ J Radiol 9: 93–95

Yuan A, Yang PC, Chang DB, Yu CJ, Kuo SH, Luh KT (1992) Lung sequestration diagnosis with ultrasound an triplex doppler technique in an adult. Chest 102: 1880–1882

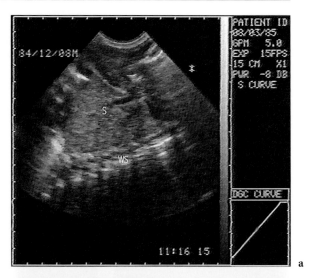

a

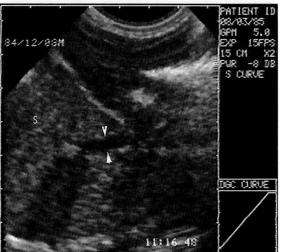

b

▶

Fig. 4.78a–c. Three-month-old boy with breathing difficulty and left thoracic swelling. Chest X-ray showed a left inferior tumor shadow with displacement of the mediastinum to the right. **a, b** Ultrasound shows a consolidation with a liver-like echo pattern over the left diaphragm; the vessels supplying this mass are depicted (*arrowheads*). *S*, Sequestration; *SC*, spinal column. **c** Angiographic confirmation of the ultrasound findings. (Case report and images by courtesy of Prof. A. Anderegg, Lausanne)

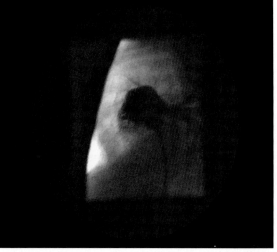

c

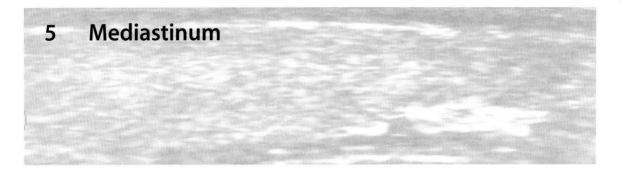

5 Mediastinum

5.1
Mediastinum – Transthoracic

W. BLANK

Sonography is usually not performed in the mediastinum. However, its application in this location can be very worthwhile. As early as in 1971, Goldberg pointed out the suprasternal sonographic access to the mediastinum. In the 1970s, the procedure was nearly forgotten outside of cardiology. In the mid-1980s, sonography of the mediastinum was researched in pediatrics (Lengerke and Schmid 1988; Liu et al. 1988), as well as in adult medicine and its efficiency was proved (Braun 1983; Heckemann 1983; Blank 1986; Wernicke 1986; Brüggemann et al. 1991). In the following years, the diagnostic potential of sonography was systematically researched (Heizel 1985; Wernicke 1986, 1991). Further possibilities were disclosed by the application of color-Doppler sonography (Betsch 1994; Dietrich et al. 1997, 1999).

Sonographic Investigation Technique and Reporting

Profound knowledge of anatomy is absolutely essential (Fig. 5.1). The investigation procedure is based on Heinzmann's stratification of the mediastinum into eight compartments, which correspond to the various lymph node groups. Because of the small sonic window, only 3.5- and 5-MHz sector, convex, and vector transducers with small apertures are suitable for sonographic diagnosis. In sonography, the mediastinum is accessed from the suprasternal and parasternal, occasionally also from the infrasternal, approach (Blank et al.

1996a). The large vessels and their spatial relationship to the heart in the various planes serve as cardinal structures. The investigation from suprasternal is performed with the patient in supine position. Viewing the upper mediastinum is facilitated by having the patient recline his head, ideally by cushioning the thoracic spine. Turning the head to the right and left is additionally helpful. In the right- and left-sided position described by Wernicke in 1998 and by Brüggemann et al. in 1991, the mediastinum is shifted and the pulmonary cavity displaced, which permits better viewing of the mediastinum. It is easier to assess the mediastinum in expiration.

Sonoanatomy

In principle, from suprasternal, the supraaortic and paratracheal regions, as well as the aorticopulmonary window, can be imaged (Fig. 5.2) (Table 5.1). For this purpose, half-sagittal (from the right and left side), coronary, and transverse images are needed. Cervical portions of the esophagus (posterior mediastinum) can also be visualized (5–8 cm) (Fig. 5.3) (Blank et al. 1998). From parasternal, the combined use of the right- and left-sided lateral decubitus position permits evaluation of the anterior and mid mediastinum. For this purpose, the transducer is placed adjacent to the sternum, cranially, and then moved caudad. Anatomical structures visualized through transverse and sagittal sections in angulated planes are summarized in Tables 5.2 and 5.3 (Figs. 5.4–5.6).

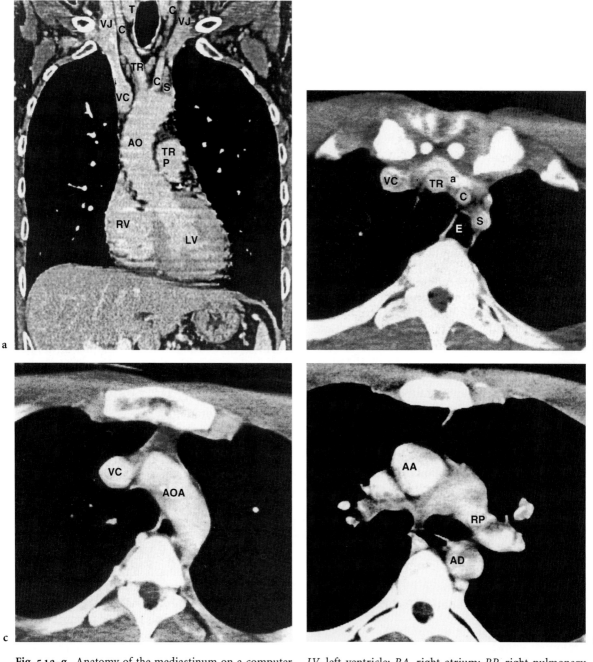

Fig. 5.1a–g. Anatomy of the mediastinum on a computer tomogram. **a** CT reconstruction of the coronary section level. **b–h** Transverse sections of the mediastinum from cranial to caudal. *a*, brachiocephalic veins; *AA*, aorta ascendens; *AD*, aorta descendens; *AO*, aorta; *AOA*, aortic arch; *C*, carotid artery; *E*, esophagus; *LP*, left pulmonary artery; *LV*, left ventricle; *RA*, right atrium; *RP*, right pulmonary artery; *RV*, right ventricle; *S*, subclavian artery; *T*, thyroid; *TP*, pulmonary trunk; *TR*, brachiocephalic trunk; *VC*, superior vena cava; *VCI*, inferior vena cava; *VJ*, jugular vein. **e–g** see p. 93

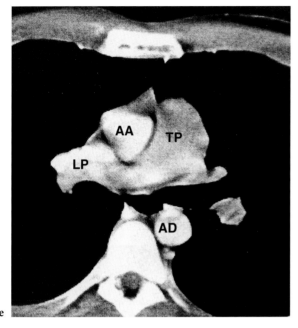
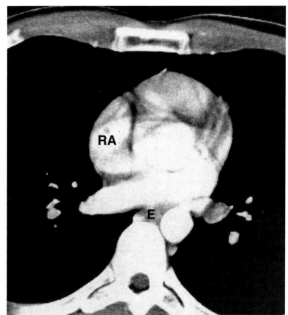

e   f

Fig. 5.1 e–g. Legend see p. 92

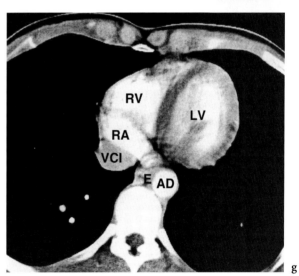

g

Table 5.1. Suprasternal access (supine position)

Superior/anterior mediastinum:
Right side – tracheal region
Brachiocephalic trunk, carotid artery,
subclavian artery
Aortic arch
Superior vena cava, brachiocephalic veins
Pulmonary trunk, pulmonary arteries
Left atrium, pulmonary veins
Thymus
Retrosternal space

Table 5.2. Parasternal access (lateral decubitus, right side)

Anterior/middle mediastinum:
Superior vena cava
Ascending aorta
Right pulmonary artery
Left atrium, pulmonary veins
Left atrium, right atrium

Table 5.3. Parasternal access (lateral decubitus, left side)

Anterior/middle mediastinum:
Descending aorta
Pulmonary trunk
Left atrium, pulmonary veins
Left ventricle, right ventricle, right atrium

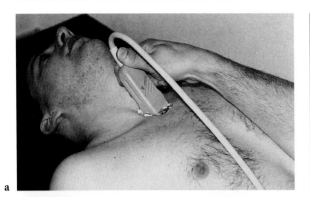

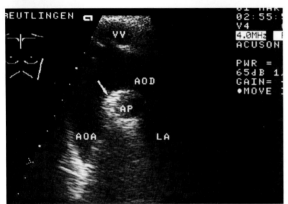

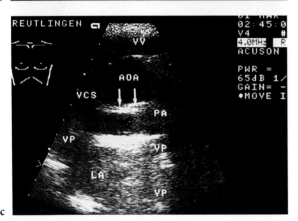

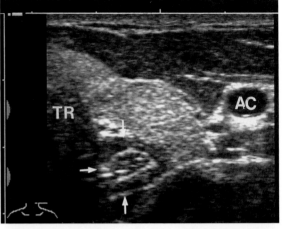

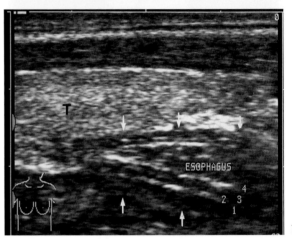

Fig. 5.3. **a** The cervical portions of the esophagus (*arrows*) show the left thyroid gland dorso-medial if the ultrasound probe is tilted slightly laterally. *TR*, trachea; *AC*, carotid artery. **b** High-resolution ultrasound probes allow a five-layer separation to be made of the esophagus wall (*arrows*). When the patient swallows, the course of the peristaltic wave and the passage of a highly reflexogenic air–liquid portion can be observed. Average wall thickness is 2.5 mm. *T*, thyroid

Fig. 5.2. **a** Suprasternal examination. The ultrasound head is located in the jugular fossa, there is a cushion under the shoulders, and the head is reclined at the maximum angle. **b** Suprasternal, sagittal section. The aortic pulmonary window (*arrow*) between the aortic arch and the pulmonary artery (*AP*) shown in the cross-section. *AOA*, ascending aorta; *AOD*, descending aorta; *LA*, left atrium; *VV*, brachiocephalic vein. **c** Suprasternal, coronary section. Lateral to the partly cut ascending aorta (*AOA*) the superior vena cava (*VCS*) leading into the brachiocephalic vein (*VV*). The aortic pulmonary window (*arrow*) between the longitudinal right pulmonary artery (*PA*) and the AOA, further in the caudal direction the left atrium (*LA*) leading to the pulmonary veins (*VP*)

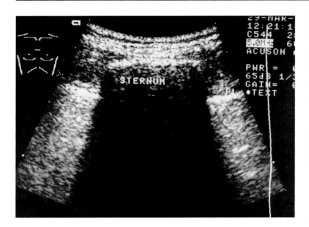

Fig. 5.4. Normal findings. Parasternal section in the supine position. The view into the mediastinum is blocked by the sternum and the inflated lung. *PL*, pleura

The infrasternal access only provides a limited view of caudal portions of the posterior mediastinum. The esophagus, aorta, and vena cava are seen at the point where they pass through the diaphragm. Transverse and sagittal images in angulated planes are obtained through the left lobe of the liver (Fig. 5.7) (Blank et al. 1996a; Janssen et al. 1997).

Imaging Compartments of the Mediastinum

The upper and mid mediastinum can be imaged well on sonography. The suprasternal access permits adequate evaluation in 90%–95% of cases. The posterior mediastinum, paravertebral region, the hilum of the lung, and the immediate retrosternal space, however, can only be partly assessed from a transthoracic approach (Table 5.4).

Table 5.4. Factors that restrict visualization of mediastinal structures

- Adiposity, large breasts
- Pulmonary emphysema
- Distortion of the mediastinum (surgery, inflammation, radiotherapy)
- Deformity of the vertebral column

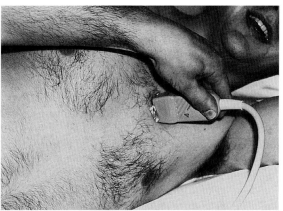

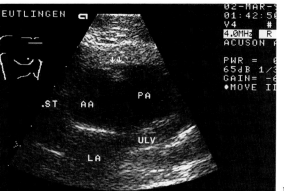

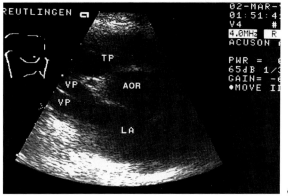

Fig. 5.5. a Parasternal examination in the left lateral position. **b** Left parasternal, transversal section. The pulmonary artery (*PA*) winds around the cross-sectional ascending aorta (*AA*). In between is the upper pericardial recess (*double arrow*), sternum (*ST*), left atrium (*LA*), upper lung veins (*ULV*). **c** Left parasternal, sagittal section. At the level of the aorta root (*AOR*) ventral crossing through the truncus pulmonalis (*TP*), dorsal left atrium (*LA*) joining pulmonary veins (*VP*)

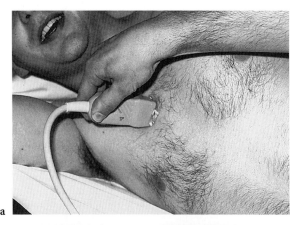

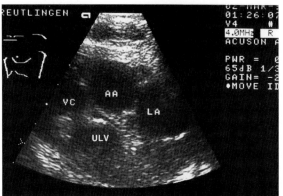

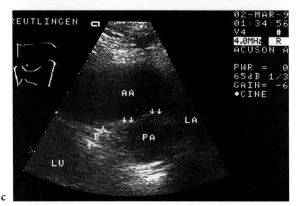

Fig. 5.6. a Parasternal examination in right lateral position. **b** Right parasternal transversal section. *AA*, ascending aorta; *VC*, superior vena cava; *LA*, left atrium; *ULV*, upper lung vein **c** Right parasternal sagittal section. A successful depiction of the ascending aorta (*AA*), the pulmonary artery (*PA*) in cross-section with the aortic pulmonary window (*double arrow*) in between, and of the subcarinal region. A bronchus (*B*) can be depicted as an echogenic reflection (*single arrow*). *LU*, lung; *LA*, left atrium

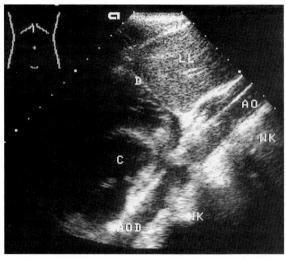

Fig. 5.7. Infrasternal sonography. Sagittal section. The esophagus (*arrow*) can be observed at the passage through the diaphragm (*D*) ventrolaterally to the aorta (*AO*). The descending aorta (*AOD*) is partly covered by artifacts. *VB*, vertebral body; *LL*, left liver lobe; *C*, cor

Imaging Tumors in the Mediastinum

Approximately 75% of clinically relevant space-occupying masses in the adult mediastinum are located in the anterior and mid mediastinum and are therefore readily accessible for sonographic assessment (Rosenberg 1983). The topographic position of a mediastinal space-occupying mass, its size, and its mobility can be determined by sonography. High-resolution sonography permits good differentiation of tissue on the basis of echogenicity (cystic, solid to calcified). Surrounding vessels can also be imaged well in the B-mode. More detailed information (invasion into vessels, tumor vascularization) can be obtained by color-Doppler sonography (Betsch 1994; Blank and Braun 1995).

Various space-occupying masses in the mediastinum have a characteristic sonomorphology (Table 5.5). A definite diagnosis, however, is usually made after removal of tissue and its histological investigation (see Sect. 5.2; Figs. 5.19 – 5.21).

Table 5.5. Sonomorphology of space-occupying masses in the mediastinum. (Modified according to Wernecke 1991)

Appearance	Type of space occupation
Anechoic	Cystic formations, vessels
Hypoechoic	Lymphomas, "active" lymph nodes, more rarely "silent" lymph nodes
Hypoechoic or inhomogeneous echoes	Carcinoma, filiae, inflammation, aneurysm
Echodense	Physiological structures, thymus, scar (exceptions: occasional liposarcomas and teratocarcinomas)

Table 5.6. Transthoracic sonography of the mediastinum

Advantages	Disadvantages
Dynamic imaging	Investigator-dependent
Free selection of sectional planes	Only parts of the mediastinum are accessible
Good imaging of the aortopulmonary window	–
Punctures: low rate of complications	Only punctures in the anterior mediastinum are possible

Diagnostic Value of Sonography, Chest Radiographs, and Computed Tomography

Sonography is superior to survey radiographs of the chest in the assessment of nearly all portions of the mediastinum (with the exception of the paravertebral region). In the evaluation of supra-aortic, pericardial, prevascular, and paratracheal regions, sonography has a sensitivity of 90%–100% and is nearly as reliable as computed tomography (CT). However, in the aorticopulmonary window and the subcarinal region, sonography achieves a sensitivity of only 82%–70% (Wernicke 1990; Brüggemann et al. 1991; Betsch 1994; Dietrich 1996). Thus, sonography occupies an intermediary position between chest radiographs and CT (Castellino et al. 1986; Bollen et al. 1994) (Table 5.6).

General Indications

Ultrasonographic investigation of the mediastinum is performed after chest radiographs have been obtained and the findings are inconclusive, or if a mediastinal space-occupying mass is suspected. Sonography is the first investigation procedure in cases of acute chest symptoms. The indications are listed in Table 5.7 (Fig. 5.8).

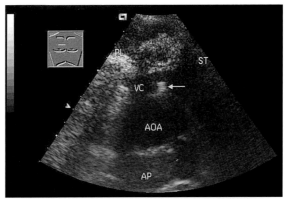

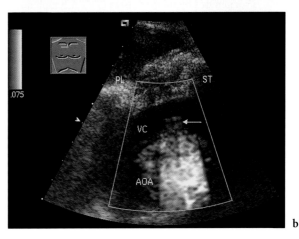

Fig. 5.8a, b. Known non-Hodgkin's lymphoma. a Acute upper inflow congestion. Condition after port implantation. B-image sonography of still parasternal tumor masses. The port catheter can be differentiated as an echogenic double structure (*arrow*) in the hypoechoic vena cava. *AOA*, ascending aorta; *AP*, right pulmonary artery; *ST*, sternum; *PL*, pleura. b Thrombosis of the vena cava superior (*VC*) can be substantiated

Table 5.7. General indications for transthoracic sonography
of the mediastinum

- Acute thoracic symptoms
- Chest radiograph: space-occupying mass
  in the mediastinum
- Chest radiograph: indefinite space-occupying mass
- Tumor staging (vascular complications)
- Monitoring the course of disease/therapy
  (tumor therapy)
- Puncture and drainage

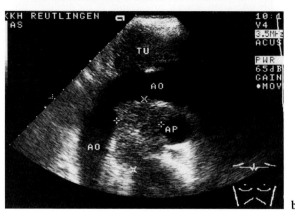

▶

Fig. 5.9 a, b. Lymph node tuberculosis. **a** Suprasternal semi-
sagittal section, right. Dorsally to the color-Doppler sonographic image of the brachiocephalic trunk (*TRBC*), one
can see a hypoechoic, indistinctly delineated lymph node
(*crosses*) in the paratracheal region, which normally has
a homogeneous, hyperechoic structure. The diagnosis of
lymph node tuberculosis was made possible by color-
Doppler sonography of the fine-needle puncture. *LU*, lung
b Suprasternal sonography in a sagittal section. The aorta
(*AO*) is surrounded by tumor masses (*TU*). A lymph node
infiltrating in the direction of the aortic arch and the pulmonary artery (*AP*) can be depicted in the aortic pulmonary window. Fine-needle puncture biopsy (0.9 mm).
Histology: metastasis of a prostate carcinoma

Specific Sonographic Findings in Selected Space-Occupying Masses in the Mediastinum

Lymph Node Disease

Based on their hypoechoic transformation,
inflamed and enlarged lymph nodes (e.g., Boeck's
disease), or lymph nodes invaded by tumor
(Hodgkin's or non-Hodgkin's lymphoma, lymph
node metastases) can be well differentiated from
the surrounding hyperechoic tissue (Figs. 5.9,
5.10). Under treatment, lymph nodes again become
increasingly echogenic (Wernicke 1991). Color-
Doppler sonography will reveal reduced blood
circulation (Betsch 1994). With the use of high-resolution devices, normal mediastinal lymph nodes
(hypoechoic) are also visualized very often (paratracheal, aorticopulmonary window). A reliable
differentiation of pathological processes, however,
is not possible (Dietrich et al. 1995, 1999).

Fig. 5.10. a Primary sonographic examination of an upper ▶
inflow congestion. Multiple lymph nodes (*LN*) suspected of
malignity in the neck region. The panorama presentation
("Sie-Scape", from Siemens) enables an impressive documentation of a relatively large region of the body. **b** Low-
echo (*arrows*) tumor infiltration into the thyroid gland.
After tumor masses (*crosses*) reaching into the retrosternal
region. **c** Left lateral parasternal section, in the vicinity
of the infiltrating low-echo mass (*crosses*). The wall of the
aorta (*AO*) can no longer be sharply delineated. *ST*, sternum;
R, rib. **d** Pericardial deposits and pericardial effusion
(*crosses*). Suspected diagnosis of bronchial carcinoma
(man, smoker) with substantiation of a mass suspected of
being a metastasis in the region of the right adrenal gland
(*crosses*). The diagnosis was confirmed by a sonographically
controlled parasternal punch biopsy (Sonocan needle,
1.2-mm diameter). Histology: small-cell bronchial carcinoma. **e** Chest X-ray overview. Mediastinal dissemination.
f Computer tomogram. Tumor on the right lower lobar
bronchus with extensive mediastinal metastases

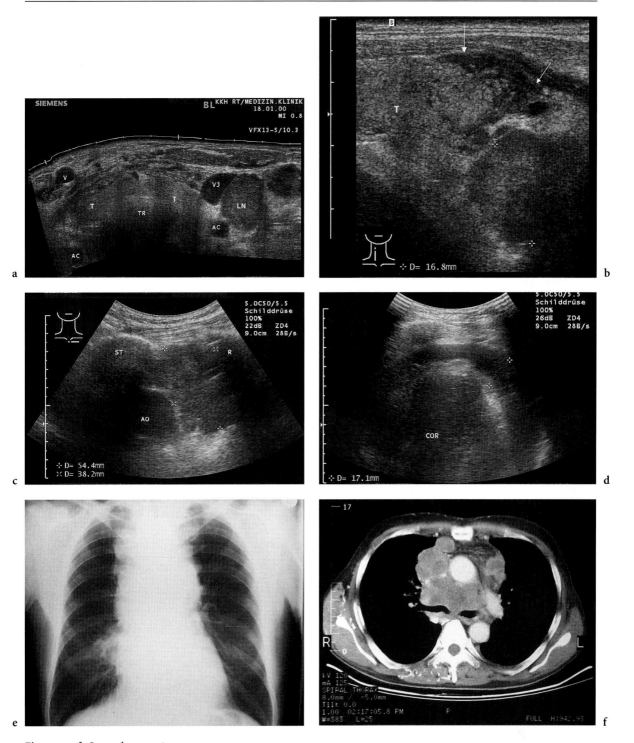

Fig. 5.10 a–f. Legend see p. 98

Tumors of the Thymus

The thymus is located in the anterior mediastinum, behind the sternum. In adults, it cannot be distinguished from its hyperechoic surroundings. Various malignant tumors may originate from the thymus; thymomas and lymphomas are the most common ones (more rarely: germ cell carcinoma, carcinoids and carcinomas). These entities have characteristic sonographic features (Fig. 5.11) (Table 5.8). The diagnosis is verified by performing a sonography- or computed tomography-guided biopsy (Schuler et al. 1995; see also Chap. 9).

Retrosternal Portions of the Thyroid and Parathyroid

These can be reliably assigned to the thyroid or the parathyroid on the basis of their topography and typical sonographic pattern. In problematic cases, color-Doppler sonography may be used to prove the source organ of the lesion.

Table 5.8. Sonomorphology of thymomas

Benign	Malignant
Hypoechoic	Hypoechoic, inhomogeneous
Sharp margins	Blurred margins
Rounded, partly lobed	Tumor cones
No infiltration	Infiltration (pericardium, vessels)

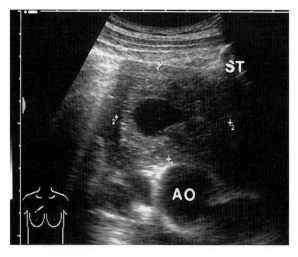

Fig. 5.11. Thymoma. Parasternal, transversal section. Even with the patient in the supine position, it was possible to see a low-echo mass in a ventral position to the aorta and well delineated. Central liquid area. Sonographically controlled incision biopsy (diameter 1.2 mm). *AO*, aorta; *ST*, sternum

Parathyroid adenomas extending retrosternally usually appear as markedly hypoechoic, oval space-occupying masses (typical laboratory constellation: increased parathyroid hormone and calcium). Punctures may be helpful to differentiate lymph node enlargement (Braun 1992).

Mediastinal Cysts

Pericardial and bronchial cysts can usually be clearly identified on the basis of their cystic character (Fig. 5.12).

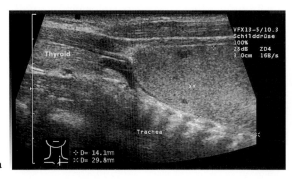

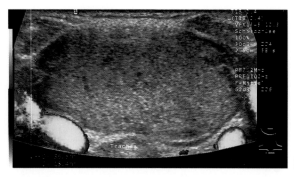

Fig. 5.12a, b. Mediastinal cysts. **a** Suprasternal sagittal section. Smooth-edged, homogeneously structured mass (*crosses*), ventral to the trachea. The proximal esophagus is recognizable dorsal to the thyroid gland on the left in the picture. **b** No blood circulation is detectable in the cross section even with this highly sensitive technology. Movement of liquid is made recognizable in the B-image and in the color Doppler sonography by a shaking movement. Diagnostic fine-needle puncture. Therapeutically operative resection due to compression syndrome

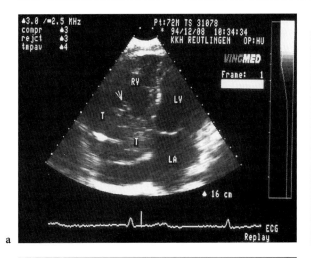

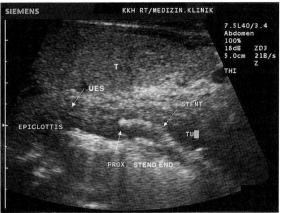

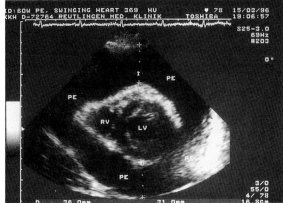

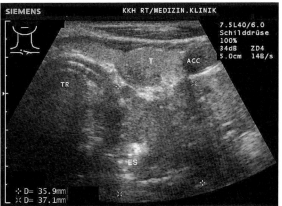

Fig. 5.13. a Chronic lymphatic leukemia affecting the right heart (*T*). As a result, tricuspid stenosis and AV block, III grade. *LA*, left atrium; *LV*, left ventricle; *RV*, right ventricle. **b** Large, chronic pericardial effusion (*PE*). (Images provided by Dr. Hust, Cardiology, Reutlingen)

Fig. 5.14. a Proximal esophageal carcinoma spreading over the wall (*TU*) with infiltration into the epiglottis, upper esophageal sphincter (*UES*, *arrow*). The overgrown metal stent (*arrow*) is well delineated. An image with plenty of contrast and low in artifacts as a result of tissue-harmonic imaging. *T*, thyroid. **b** Tumor masses (*crosses*) with infiltration and stenosis of the esophagus (*ES*)

Changes in the Pericardium

Such changes include pericardial effusion, hematopericardium, and tumor invasion (Fig. 5.13).

Esophageal Disease

Proximal and distal portions of the esophagus can be clearly visualized by the suprasternal and infrasternal access. Esophageal tumors crossing the wall are seen as hypoechoic tumor formations with blurred margins (Fig. 5.14). In cases of surgical replacement of the esophagus, the upper anas-

tomosis can be viewed. Recurrent tumors can also be detected (Blank et al. 1998) (Fig. 5.15).
Sonography is a valuable aid in the detection of "dysphagia close to the cardia" (Blank et al. 1996a; Janssen et al. 1997).

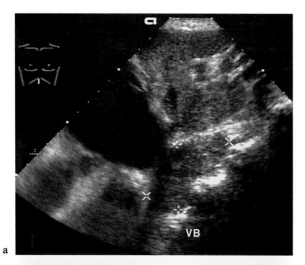

a

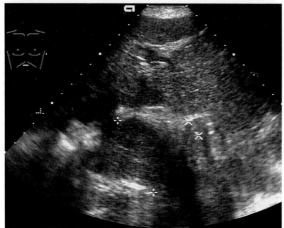

b

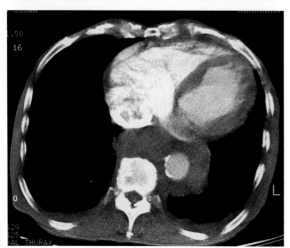

c

Fig. 5.15a–c. Extensive esophageal carcinoma. **a** Clinical dysphagia. Endoscopic distal esophageal stenosis. No tumor could be established with certainty by biopsy. Sonography with infrasternal, sagittal section of the tumor formation lying ventrally to the spinal column (posterior mediastinum). *VB*, vertebral body. **b** Tumor (*crosses*) located infrasternally in transversal section at the distal esophagus (*large crosses*) cannot be delineated. Percutaneously controlled transhepatic fine-needle cut biopsy (Sonocan, 0.9 mm). Histology: esophageal carcinoma. **c** Computer tomography. Mass in the posterior mediastinum surrounding the descending aorta

◀

Summary

Mediastinal space-occupying masses are most frequently found in the anterior upper mediastinum. They can be evaluated with transthoracic sonography nearly as reliably as with CT.

The disadvantages of sonography, however, are significant. The procedure is strongly investigator-dependent and only reveals portions of the mediastinum compared to CT. Moreover, the image quality is highly variable. These disadvantages can be balanced by the application of endoluminal transesophageal and endobronchial sonography (see Sect. 5.2 and Chap. 6).

Acknowledgments. I would like to express my thanks to Professor-Dr. Lenz (chief consultant surgeon in the Radiology Department of the Steinenberg Clinic, Reutlingen) for preparing and providing the radiological findings, and to Mr. Klinkmüller and my son Valentin for the technical photographic work.

References

Betsch B (1994) Farbdopplersonographie des Mediastinums. Radiologe 34:599–604

Betsch B, Knopp MV, van Kaick G (1992) Malignant tumors and lymphomas of the mediastinum: Diagnosis and follow-up with color assisted doppler sonography. Eur J Cancer Res Clin Oncol 118:107

Betsch B, Berndt R, Knopp MV, Schmähl A, Trost U, Delorme S (1994) Vergleich von Computertomographie und B-Bild-Sonographie in der bildgebenden Diagnostik des Mediastinums. Bildgebung 61:295–298

Blank W, Braun B (1995) Gewebsdiagnostik durch Dopplersonographie. Bildgebung 62:31–35

Blank W, Braun B, Gekeler E (1986) Ultraschalldiagnostik und Feinnadelpunktion pleuraler, pulmonaler und mediastinaler Prozesse. In: Hansmann M (Hrsg) Ultraschalldiagnostik. Springer, Berlin Heidelberg New York Tokyo, S 562–565

Blank W, Braun B, Schuler A, Wild K (1996a) Die percutane Sonographie zur Differenzierung der Dysphagie. Ultraschall Med (Suppl. 1):32

Blank W, Schuler A, Wild K, Braun B (1996b) Transthoracic sonography of the mediastinum. Eur J Ultrasound 3:179–190

Blank W, Schwaiger U, Wild K, Braun B (1998) Die percutane Sonographie zur Darstellung des cervicalen Ösophagus. Ultraschall Med (Suppl. 1):4

Bollen EC, Goci R, v Hofgrootenboer BE, Versteege CWM, Engelshove HA, Lamers RJ (1994) Interobserver variability and accuracy of computed tomographic assessment of nodal status in lung cancer. Ann Thorax Surg 58:158–162

Braun B (1983) Abdominelle und thorakale Ultraschalldiagnostik. In: Bock HE (Hrsg) Klinik der Gegenwart. Urban & Schwarzenberg, München, S 1141–1145

Braun B (1992) Schilddrüse. In: Braun B, Günther R, Schwerk WB (Hrsg) Ultraschalldiagnostik. Lehrbuch und Atlas. ecomed, Landsberg/Lech, III-3.1

Brüggemann A, Greie A, Lepsien G (1991) Real-time-sonography of the mediastinum in adults: a study in 100 healthy volunteers. Surg Endosc 5:150–153

Castellino RA, Blank N, Hoppe RT et al. (1986) Hodgkin disease: contributions of chest CT in the initial staging evaluation. Radiology 160:603–605

Dietrich CF, Liesen M, Wehrmann T, Caspary WF (1995) Mediastinalsonographie: Eine neue Bewertung der Befunde. Ultraschall Med 16:61

Dietrich CF, Liesen M, Buhl R, Herrmann G, Kirchner I, Caspary WF, Wehrmann T (1997) Detection of normal mediastinal lymphnodes by ultrasonography. Acta Radiol 38:965–969

Dietrich CF, Chickakli M, Burgon I, Wehrmann T, Wiewrodt R, Buhl R, Caspary WF (1999) Mediastinal lymphnodes demonstrated by mediastinal sonography: Activity marker in patients with cystic fibrosis. J Clin Ultrasound 27:9–14

Goldberg GG (1971) Suprasternal ultrasonography. JAMA 15:245–250

Heckemann R (1983) Sonographische Tumordiagnostik im Mediastinum. Therapiewoche 33:123–137

Heitzmann EK (1988) The mediastinum. Springer, Berlin, Heidelberg, New York

Heizel M (1985) Sonographische Topographie des oberen vorderen Mediastinums. Ultraschall 6:101–109

Janssen J, Johanns W, Lehnhardt M, Jakobeit C, Greiner L (1997) Die transkutane Sonographie des gastroösophagealen Übergangs im prospektiven Vergleich mit der Endoskopie. Dtsch Med Wochenschr 122:1167–1171

v. Lengerke HV, Schmid HC (1988) Mediastinalsonographie im Kindesalter. Radiologe 28:460–465

Liu P, Daneman A, Stringer DA (1988) Real-time-sonography of mediastinal and juxtamediastinal masses in infants and children. J Can Assoc Radiol 39:198–203

Rosenberg JC (1993) Neoplasms of the mediastinum. In: De Vita VT, Hellman S, Rosenberg SA (eds) Cancer: principles & practice of oncology. Lippincott, Philadelphia, pp 759–775

Schuler A, Blank W, Braun B (1995) Sonographisch-interventionelle Diagnostik bei Thymomen. Ultraschall Med 16:62

Wernecke K, Peters PE, Galanski M (1986) Mediastinal tumors: evaluation of suprasternal sonographie. Radiology 159:405–409

Wernecke K, Pötter R, Peters PE (1988) Parasternal mediastinal sonography: Sensitivity in the detection of anterior mediastinal and subcarinal tumors. Am J Roentgenol 150:1021–1026

Wernecke K (1991) Mediastinale Sonographie, Untersuchungstechnik, diagnostische Effizienz und Stellenwert in der bildgebenden Diagnostik des Mediastinums. Springer, Berlin Heidelberg, New York Tokyo

Wernecke K, Peters PE, Galanski M (1986) Mediastinal tumors: evaluation of suprasternal sonography. Radiology 159:405–409

5.2
Mediastinum – Transesophageal

J. T. ANNEMA, M. VESELIC, K. F. RABE

The analysis of mediastinal masses, for example enlarged mediastinal lymph nodes in patients with lung cancer, is of major clinical importance. Histologic proof of the diagnosis often requires invasive procedures such as mediastinoscopy or mediastinotomy, thoracoscopy, or even thoracotomy. These procedures are not only burdensome for patients, but they also have limitations in their reach, require hospitalization, and are therefore accompanied with high costs. The development of endoscopic ultrasound (EUS) has opened up new diagnostic possibilities. This technique is currently established as a diagnostic tool in the staging of specific gastrointestinal neoplasms. Since 1995, transesophageal endoscopic ultrasound has also been performed in pulmonary medicine in order to establish a diagnosis for mediastinal lesions and to stage the mediastinum in patients with lung cancer (Giovanni et al. 1995; Pedersen et al. 1996). The central position of the esophagus in the posterior mediastinum provides good access to this region.

The Technique

Transesophageal endoscopic ultrasound is performed with devices which are used in the gastroenterology practice. Currently, there are both radial and linear ultrasound probes available. EUS enables an anatomical visualization of the esophagus and its surrounding structures. It is possible to obtain tissue samples of lesions which lie adjacent to the esophagus by puncturing the target lesion under ultrasound guidance. The material obtained in this way is suitable for cytological as well as molecular-biologic diagnosis, for example, polymerase chain reaction (PCR) analysis for mycobacterium tuberculosis.

For transesophageal *endoscopic ultrasound-guided fine needle aspiration* biopsy (EUS-FNA), only a linear ultrasound probe is used. The procedure is performed in an ambulant setting and does not require any specific preparations. The patient is positioned in the left lateral position and, after spraying a local anesthetic to the pharynx, the procedure is performed under conscious sedation. The ultrasound probe is advanced into the distal part of the esophagus until the left lobe of the liver is visualized. From this landmark, the scoop is stepwise withdrawn whilst making circular movements enabling the investigator to visualize most parts of the mediastinum. Location, size, and echo features of lesions are determined. It is recommended that these findings be recorded and stored.

The registered lymph nodes are anatomically classified according to the Naruke classification (Mountain and Dressler 1997; Fig. 5.16). Suspicious lesions can be punctured smoothly through the wall of the esophagus under real-time ultrasound guidance. An on-site evaluation of the punctured material by a cytologist is recommended. In the hands of an experienced investigator, EUS-FNA of the mediastinum takes about 30 min to perform.

There are no absolute *contraindications* for an endoscopic investigation of the upper gastrointestinal tract, although esophagus strictures and diverticula display an increased risk of perforation. In gastroenterology examinations, especially when the pancreas is punctured, complication rates of EUS-FNA are between 0.5 and 2% (Giovanni et al. 1995; Gress et al. 1997b; Wiersema 1997; Williams et al. 1999). There are no complications reported so far in the investigation of the mediastinum with EUS-FNA (Fritscher-Ravens et al. 1999, 2000; Hühnerbein et al. 1998; Janssen et al. 1998; Rabe et al. 1998; Silvestri et al. 1996).

The theoretical *advantages* of this new diagnostic procedure – as compared to radiological and surgical alternatives – are numerous (Table 5.9). EUS-FNA is more sensitive in the determination of mediastinal lymph nodes as compared to chest CT (Hawes 1994), and enables a real-time controlled

Table 5.9. EUS-FNA: advantages and limitations

Advantages	Limitations
Minimally invasive	Para- and pretracheal lymph nodes
Real-time puncture	Operator dependency
Safe	
Highly cost-effective	

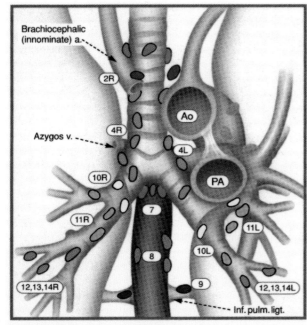

Superior Mediastinal Nodes

- 1 Highest Mediastinal
- 2 Upper Paratracheal
- 3 Pre-vascular and Retrotracheal
- 4 Lower Paratracheal (including Azygos Nodes)

N_2 = single digit, ipsilateral
N_3 = single digit, contralateral or supraclavicular

Aortic Nodes

- 5 Subaortic (A-P window)
- 6 Para-aortic (ascending aorta or phrenic)

Inferior Mediastinal Nodes

- 7 Subcarinal
- 8 Paraesophageal (below carina)
- 9 Pulmonary Ligament

N_1 Nodes

- 10 Hilar
- 11 Interlobar
- 12 Lobar
- 13 Segmental
- 14 Subsegmental

Fig. 5.16 a, b. Lymph node classification for lung cancer staging. (From Mountain and Dressler 1997)

puncture. In comparison with the surgical alternatives, EUS-FNA is less invasive, it is performed on an outpatient basis, and is more *cost-effective* (Gress et al. 1997a).

Limitations of EUS-FNA are located in the pre- and paratracheal areas, while air in the trachea and main bronchi disturbs the ultrasound waves. In assessing the mediastinum, mediastinoscopy and EUS-FNA are partly complementary. Mediastinoscopy provides good access to the pre- and paratracheal lymph node stations, whereas EUS-FNA is more suitable in assessing the subcarinal and paraesophageal lymph nodes, as well as lymph nodes in the aorta pulmonary window and the ligamentum pulmonale (Fig. 5.16; Bhutani 2000, Serna et al. 1998).

Table 5.10. EUS-FNA: mediastinal lymph nodes

Author	Patients (n)	Diagnostic accuracy (%)
Giovannini et al. 1995	22	83
Silvestri et al. 1996	27	89
Gress et al. 1997	43	95
Wiersema et al. 1997	192[a]	92
Janssen et al. 1998	35	91
Rabe et al. 1998	95	80
Williams et al. 1999	82	90
Fritscher-Ravens 2000	35	97

[a] Data include all gastrointestinal lymph nodes.

Clinical Implications

For the analysis of mediastinal lymph nodes, a EUS procedure without obtaining biopsies is of limited value. Neither size nor ultrasound characteristics are able to accurately define malignant infiltration of lymph nodes or other lesions (Bhutani et al. 1997). It is established that EUS-FNA has a high diagnostic accuracy (80%–97%; Table 5.10) in the assessment of mediastinal lymph nodes (Fritscher-Ravens et al. 2000; Giovanni et al. 1995; Gress et al. 1997a, b; Hühnerbein et al. 1998; Janssen et al. 1998; Rabe et al. 1998; Silvestri et al. 1996; Wiersema et al. 1997; Williams et al. 1999).

The current treatment strategy for bronchial carcinoma is based on histological assessment and tumor spread. In the future, there may be an important role for EUS-FNA in the diagnosis of mediastinal lesions, especially those which are difficult, or impossible, to reach by mediastinoscopy (Bhutani 2000; Serna et al. 1998; Fig. 5.17). EUS-FNA is a valuable diagnostic technique in patients with a intrapulmonary lesion and enlarged mediastinal lymph nodes in which bronchoscopy failed to establish a diagnosis (Fritscher-Ravens et al. 1999, Fig. 5.18).

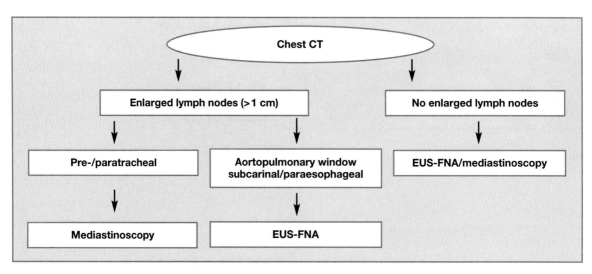

Fig. 5.17. EUS-FNA – Mediastinal staging of non-small cell lung cancer (proposal)

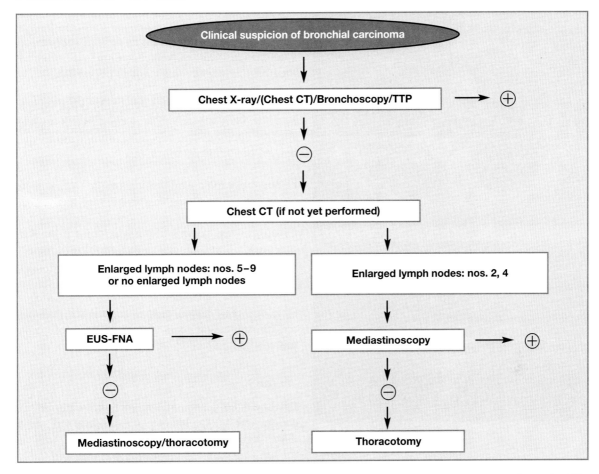

Fig. 5.18. EUS-FNA – Procedure in the case of suspected lung cancer (proposal). ⊕, Diagnosis; ⊖, no diagnosis; *TTP*, transthoracic puncture; *, optional

Case Reports

Case 1

History. A 46-year-old patient with an adenocarcinoma in the right upper lobe who is otherwise in good clinical condition.

Chest CT (Fig. 5.19 a). Mass (3 × 4 × 6 cm) in the right upper lobe, enlarged inhomogeneous subcarinal lymph node (2 × 3 × 3 cm).

Endosonography (Fig. 5.19 b). Enlarged lymph node between esophagus and the left atrium with hypoechogenic areas and irregular boundaries (lymph node station 7). In the upper right corner, the puncture needle is visible.

Cytology (Fig. 5.19 c). Large adenocarcinoma cells with vacuoles and enlarged red central nuclei. On the right side of the picture, squamous cells of the esophagus are visible.

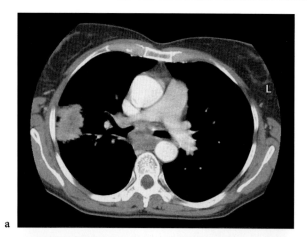

a

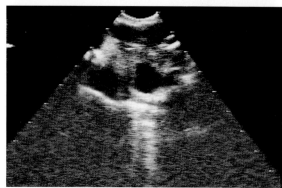

b

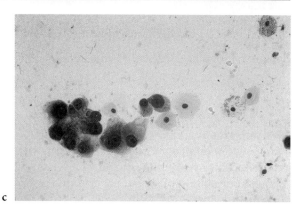

c

Fig. 5.19. **a** Chest CT. **b** EUS-FNA subcarinal lymph node. **c** Cytology: adenocarcinoma

Case 2

History. A 60-year-old housewife with a wheezing sound on respiration. A mastectomy had been performed 7 years previously due to breast cancer.

Chest CT (Fig. 5.20 a). Enlarged subcarinal lymph node (1 × 2.5 × 1 cm). The esophagus is visible slightly dorsal of the subcarinal lymph node and behind the left main bronchus.

Endosonography. An identical image to that seen on endoscopy in Case 1 was visible (see Fig. 5.19 b).

Cytology (Fig. 5.20 b). Metastasis from a lobular carcinoma. Small groups as well as solitary malignant cells with small irregular nuclei and little cytoplasm are presented.

Cytology (Fig. 5.20 c). Estrogen receptor staining confirms the diagnosis of mammary carcinoma metastasis.

Case 3

History. A 69-year-old housewife with a persistent cough and a long history of smoking. On chest X-ray, a mass is visible in the right upper lobe of the lung and the right diaphragm is elevated.

Chest CT (Fig. 5.21 a). Relatively smoothly defined intrapulmonary lesion in the right upper lobe (3 × 3 × 6 cm) closely related to the mediastinum. The esophagus is situated left retrotracheally.

Endosonography (Fig. 5.21 b). Lesion with a slight inhomogeneous structure and an irregular border with an amplified ultrasound reflex. The image is consistent with a tumor mass surrounded by compromised lung tissue. The aspiration cytology was taken from the primary tumor.

Cytology (Fig. 5.21 c). Cells of an undifferentiated large cell carcinoma. The cells contain large nuclei with an abnormal chromatin pattern. The cytoplasm is clearly defined.

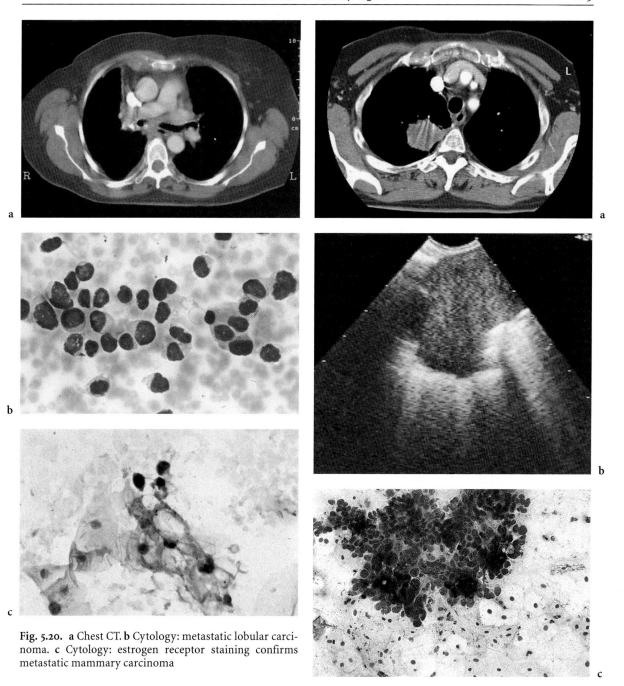

Fig. 5.20. a Chest CT. b Cytology: metastatic lobular carcinoma. c Cytology: estrogen receptor staining confirms metastatic mammary carcinoma

Fig. 5.21. a Chest CT. b EUS-FNA intrapulmonary lesion. c Cytology: undifferentiated large cell carcinoma

Case 4

History. A 57-year-old patient with severe complaints of tiredness and retrosternal pain.

Chest CT (Fig. 5.22 a). Multiple enlarged mediastinal lymph nodes in the mediastinum. Retrotracheally is the esophagus clearly visible.

Endosonography (Fig. 5.22 b). Conglomerate of enlarged lymph nodes with septation. In the bottom left corner, part of the left atrium is visible, and on the bottom right part of the pulmonary trunk.

Cytology (Fig. 5.22 c). This lymph node consists of a typical granuloma without central necrosis.

Cytology (Fig. 5.22 d). Granulomas with some lymphocytes and small groups of squamous cells from the esophagus.

Case 5

History. A 53-year-old patient with an osteosarcoma of the right tibia. A mediastinal lesion was depicted on a screening CT performed for staging purposes.

Chest CT (Fig. 5.23 a). Lesion with smooth borders (2 × 1 × 1 cm) situated in the posterior mediastinum. The heart and descending aorta are clearly depicted.

Endosonography (Fig. 5.23 b). Remarkable hypoechogenic structure situated next to the esophagus, on color Doppler ultrasound, the fluid signs are absent. The aspirate from this location is graywhite mucus.

Cytology (Fig. 5.23 c). Bronchogenic cyst. Large group of squamous cells from the esophagus in an amorphous area of mucus. In the left upper corner, bronchial epithelial cells are visible.

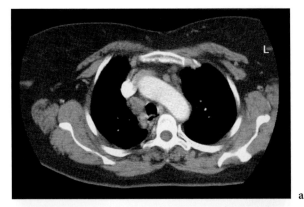

a

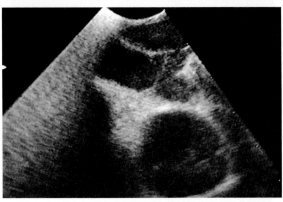

b

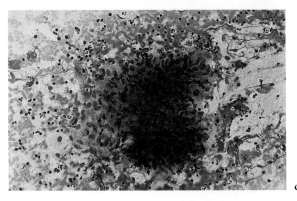

c

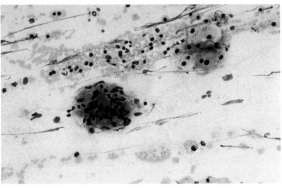

d

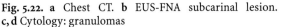

Fig. 5.22. a Chest CT. **b** EUS-FNA subcarinal lesion. **c, d** Cytology: granulomas

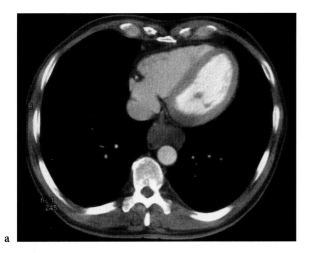

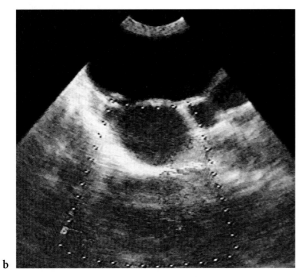

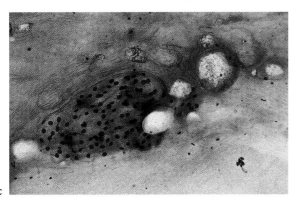

Fig. 5.23. a Chest CT. **b** EUS-FNA subcarinal anechogenic lesion. **c** Cytology: bronchogenic cyst

Summary and Future Perspectives

Up until now, EUS studies concentrated on the performance of the technique itself, the description of normal and pathological findings, and the diagnostic accuracy of EUS-FNA in the assessment of mediastinal lymph nodes. According to these studies, EUS-FNA appears to be especially suitable for the analysis of subcarinal lymph nodes and lymph nodes located in the aortopulmonary window (Bhutani 2000). Future studies are required to prospectively assess the value of EUS-FNA in comparison with current diagnostic techniques, for example mediastinoscopy. In addition to diagnostic accuracy, cost efficiency of the various diagnostic procedures and patient preference should be taken into account. These studies are required to define a place for this new, fascinating diagnostic technique in clinical practice. Currently, the application of EUS-FNA in pulmonary medicine is in the hands of a few committed investigators.

References

Bhutani MS (2000) Transesophageal endoscopic ultra-sound-guided mediastinal lymph node aspiration. Chest 117: 298 – 301

Bhutani MS, Haws RH, Hoffman BJ (1997) A comparison of the accuracy of echo features during endoscopic ultrasound (EUS) and EUS-guided fine-needle aspiration for diagnosis of malignant lymph node invasion. Gastrointest Endosc 45: 474 – 479

Fritscher-Ravens A, Petrasch S, Reinacher-Schick A, Graeven U, Konig M, Schmiegel W (1999) Diagnostic value of endoscopic ultrasonography guided fine needle aspiration cytology of mediastinal masses in patients with intrapulmonary lesions and nondiagnostic bronchoscopy. Respiration 66: 150 – 155

Fritscher-Ravens A, Soehendra N, Schirrow L, Parupudi WJS, Meyer A, Hauber HP, Pforte A (2000) Role of transesophageal endosonography-guided fine-needle aspiration in the diagnosis of lung cancer. Chest 117: 339 – 345

Giovanni M, Seitz J, Monges G, Perrier H, Rabbio I (1995) Fine-needle aspiration cytology guided by endoscopic ultrasonography: results in 141 patients. Endoscopy 127: 171 – 177

Gress FG, Hawes R, Savides T, Ikenberry S, Lehmann GA (1997a) Endoscopic ultrasound-guided fine-needle aspiration biopsy using linear array and radial scanning endosonography. Gastrointest Endosc 145: 243 – 250

Gress FG, Savides T, Sandler A et al. (1997b) Endoscopic ultrasonography, fine needle aspiration biopsy guided by endoscopic ultrasonography, and computer tomography in the preoperative staging of non-small-cell lung cancer: a comparison study. Ann Intern Med 127:604–612

Hawes RH (1994) Endoscopic ultrasound versus computed tomography in the evaluation of the mediastinum in patients with non-small cell lung cancer: a comparison study. Endoscopy 26:784–877

Hühnerbein M, Ghadimi BM, Haensch W, Schlag PM (1998) Transesophageal biopsy of mediastinal and pulmonary tumors by means of endoscopic ultrasound guidance. J Thorac Cardiovasc Surg 116:554–559

Janssen J, Johanns W, Luis W, Greiner L (1998) Clinical value of endoscopic ultrasound guided transesophageal fine needle puncture of mediastinal lesions. Dtsch Med Wochenschr 123:1402–1409

Mountain CF, Dressler CM (1997) Regional lymph node classification for lung cancer staging. Chest 111:1718–1723

Pedersen BH, Vilmann P, Folker K, Jacobsen GK, Krasnik M, Milman N, Hancke S (1996) Endoscopic ultrasonography and real-time guided fine-needle aspiration biopsy of solid lesions of the mediastinum suspected of malignancy. Chest 110:539–544

Rabe KF, Welker L, Magnussen H (1998) Endoscopic ultrasonography (EUS) of the mediastinum: safety, specificity, and results of cytology. Eur Respir J 12:974

Serna DL, Aryan HE, Chang KJ, Brenner M, Tran LM, Chen JC (1998) An early comparison between endoscopic ultrasound-guided fine-needle aspiration and mediastinoscopy for the diagnosis of mediastinal malignancy. Am Surg 64:1014–1018

Silvestri GA, Hoffman BJ, Bhutani MS, Haws RH, Coppage L, Sanders-Cliette AS, Reed CE (1996) Endoscopic ultrasound with fine needle aspiration in the diagnosis and staging of lung cancer. Ann Thorac Surg 61:1441–1446

Wiersema MJ, Vilmann P, Giovannini M, Chang KJ, Wiersema LM (1997) Endosonography-guided fine-needle aspiration biopsy: diagnostic accuracy and complication assessment. Gastroenterology 112:1087–1095

Williams DB, Sahai AV, Aabakken L et al. (1999) Endoscopic ultrasound-guided fine-needle aspiration biopsy: a large single centre experience. Gut 44:720–726

6 Endobronchial Ultrasound

F. Herth, H. D. Becker

Radiologic imaging has been proven to be unreliable in the diagnosis of mediastinal lymph nodes (Buelzebruck et al. 1992; Layer and van Kaick 1990). The view of the endoscopist, however, is limited to the lumen and the internal surface of the airways. Processes within the airway wall and outside the airways can only be assessed by indirect signs. In addition, many processes also involve the parabronchial structures. Particularly in malignancies, this can be of decisive importance for the fate of the patient. Therefore, expanding the endoscopist's view beyond the airways is essential (Becker 1995). External mediastinal thoracic ultrasound is insufficient for imaging of the paratracheal and hilar structures. With endoesophageal ultrasound (EUS), the pretracheal region and the hilar structures are inaccessible due to limited contact and interposition of the airways. It is for this reason that we have been investigating the application of endobronchial ultrasound (EBUS) since 1989 (Fig. 6.1; Becker and Herth 1999).

6.1
Instruments and Technique

Instruments used for gastrointestinal application cannot be applied inside the airways because of their diameter. Prototypes of dedicated endoscopes with an integrated curvilinear electronic transducer at the tip have not as yet been routinely applied (Ono et al. 1994). Preliminary tests using miniaturized endovascular sonographic probes did not yield useful clinical results and were aborted after a while (Huerter and Hanrath 1990). For application inside the central airways, therefore, we developed flexible catheters for the Olympus probes with a balloon tip allowing circular contact for the ultrasound, providing a complete 360° image of the parabronchial and paratracheal structures. Since the balloon provides enhancement of the ultrasound, penetration of the waves produced by 20-MHz probes is increased. Thus, under favorable conditions, structures at a dis-

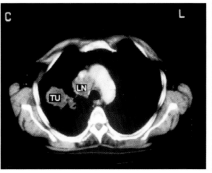 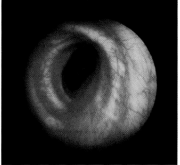 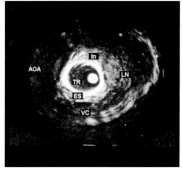

a
b
c

Fig. 6.1a–c. Exclusion of infiltration of the tracheal wall. **a** Infiltration by tumor on CT. *TU*, tumor; *LN*, lymph node. **b** Endoscopy infiltration can not be excluded. **c** Exclusion of infiltration by EBUS. *AOA*, ascending aorta; *TR*, trachea; *ES*, esophagus; *VC*, vertebral column; *ln*, small lymphode; *LN*, lymph node

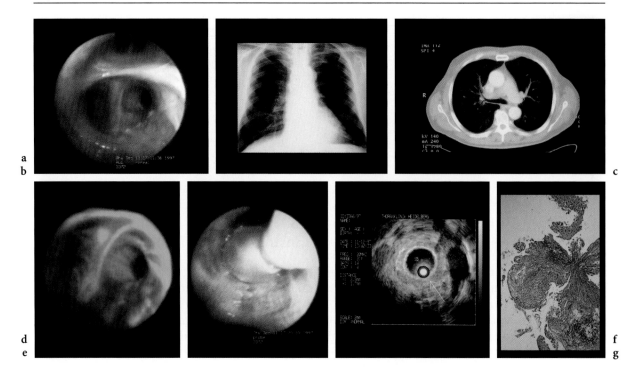

Fig. 6.2a–g. Local staging of early lung cancer. **a** Radiologically invisible tumor in right upper lobe bronchus. **b, c** Chest X-ray and CT are normal. **d** Extensive extinction of autofluorescence. **e** EBUS probe in situ. **f** Destruction of bronchial wall. **g** Biopsy proves squamous cell lung cancer

tance of up to 5 cm can be visualized. These probes have been on the market since 1999 and can be applied with standard flexible endoscopes with a biopsy channel of at least 2.6 mm. Even complete obstruction of the trachea is tolerated under local anesthesia for up to 2.5 min after sufficient preoxygenation and sedation, sufficient time to acquire diagnostic images.

6.2
Sonographic Anatomy

The wall of the central airways shows a seven-layer structure which can only be demonstrated by high magnification. The layers correspond to the mucosa and submucosa, the three layers of the cartilage, and the adjacent external structures of loose and dense connective tissue, respectively. Under low power magnification and in the periphery, only a three-layer structure is visible. Orientation using ultrasound within the mediastinum is difficult, not only due to the complex mediastinal

anatomy and motion artifacts caused by pulsation and respiration, but also due to the unusual planes of the ultrasonic images since the course of the airways has to be followed with the probes. For orientation, therefore, analyzing characteristic anatomical structures is more reliable than observing the position of the ultrasound probe inside the airway. Vessels can be diagnosed by their pulsation. But even after application of echo contrast media, identifying venous and arterial vessels can be difficult due to the great number of variations. However, since pulse oximetry is applied during the procedure, arterial pulsations can be diagnosed according to their synchronism with the acoustic signal. Lymph nodes and solid structures can be distinguished down to the size of a few millimeters from blood vessels by their higher echodensity.

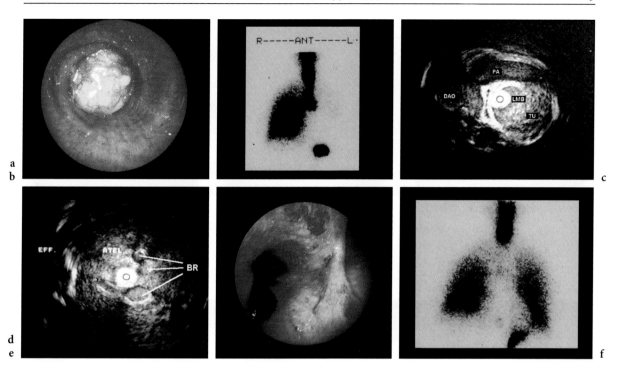

Fig. 6.3 a–f. Local staging of advanced lung cancer. **a** Occlusion of the left main bronchus by tumor. **b** Loss of perfusion and ventilation in scintigraphy. **c** Bronchial occlusion and patent pulmonary artery. *PA*, pulmonary artery; *DAO*, descending aorta; *LMB*, left main bronchus; *TU*, tumor. **d** Atelectasis (*ATEL*) and pleural effusion (*EFF*); bronchi patent (*BR*) and filled with fluid. **e** Patency of the bronchus after laser ablation. **f** Restored ventilation and perfusion

6.3
Results of Clinical Application

Tumor Staging

In the case of small, radiologically invisible tumors, the decision to carry out a local endoscopic therapeutic intervention is dependent on the intraluminal and intramural extent of the tumors within the different layers of the wall. On endobronchial ultrasound, even very small tumors of a few millimeters can be analyzed and distinguished from benign lesions and today has become the basis for curative endobronchial treatment of malignancies (Miyazu et al. 2001; Fig. 6.2). EBUS also provides important data for the decision-making process regarding endobronchial therapy in advanced lung cancer. In the case of complete bronchial obstruction, the base and surface of the tumor can be assessed, as well as whether the different layers of the bronchial wall are involved, the extent to which the tumor penetrates into the mediastinal structures, and whether the airways beyond the stenosis are patent (Fig. 6.3). Also, patency of the adjacent pulmonary artery can be established. It is important for a preoperative diagnosis to establish to what extent the great vessels such as the aorta, vena cava, and main pulmonary arteries, as well as the esophageal wall, are involved, data which is often impossible to obtain using radiological methods (Fig. 6.4). Under favorable conditions, lymph nodes can be identified down to a size of 2–3 mm and the internal structure (sinuses and folliculi), as well as small lymph vessels, can be analyzed (Shannon et al. 1996). Using endosonographic localization, the accuracy of transbronchial needle aspiration (TBNA) can be increased to as much as 90 % (Fig. 6.5).

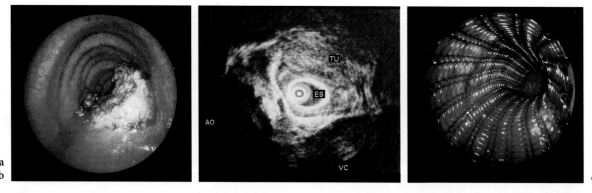

Fig. 6.4a–c. EBUS in interventional bronchoscopy. **a** Tracheal tumor after partial laser ablation. **b** Infiltration of anterior esophageal wall. *AO*, aorta; *ES*, esophagus; *TU*, tumor; *VC*, vertebral column. **c** Palliative stent insertion before external radiation due to risk of esophagotracheal fistula

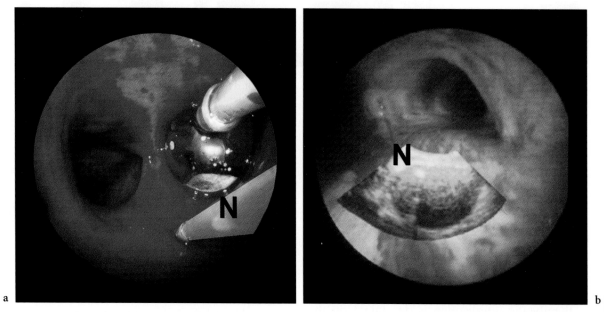

Fig. 6.5.a, b. EBUS-guided transbronchial needle aspiration of lymph nodes (*TBNA*). **a** TBNA under EBUS control. *N*, needle. **b** Echo of needle (*N*) inside lymph node

Mediastinal Masses. Mediastinal masses can only be analyzed and approached using EBUS for transtracheal and transbronchial needle biopsy if they are in direct contact with the wall of the central airways or if a great vessel is providing an acoustic window. However, for the investigation of retrosternal masses or the dorsal mediastinum, EBUS penetration is insufficient.

Great Vessels. Great vessels in the vicinity of the central airways are easily visualized due to their pulsation and low echo density. Diagnosis of tumor infiltration is also essential. Stenosis of the central airways by compression due to vascular malformations is not uncommon in early childhood. Diagnosis of thromboembolic complications of the venous system is more difficult using EBUS than using EUS. It is sometimes possible to identify pulmonary embolism by means of endobronchial or endoesophageal ultrasound, a procedure which is not usually undertaken on suspicion of pulmonary embolism.

Intrapulmonary Lesions. Intrapulmonary lesions can be easily differentiated from lung tissue. By analyzing their internal structure, we might be able to predict the histology of such lesions in the future. In atelectasis, peribronchial obstruction by lymph nodes and tumor masses can be differentiated from compression by pleural effusion or pleural masses.

Endoesophageal Application. We also applied the miniaturized probes inside the esophagus to evaluate the mediastinal lymph nodes. Obviously, penetration of the ultrasound is limited by the 20-MHz probes. Sometimes, however, lymph nodes in the aorto-pulmonary window can be visualized more clearly. Intramural lesions of the esophageal wall, such as leiomyoma and intramural diverticulosis, could also be diagnosed and differentiated from malignant lesions.

Guidance and Control of Therapeutic Interventions

EBUS is useful for exploring central airway stenosis to assess the cause and extent of the disease and to make the correct therapeutic decision such as mechanical dilatation, laser ablation, or stent implantation, as well as endoscopic control of the results. Particularly when decision-making in potentially curative endobronchial therapy of malignancies, such as photodynamic therapy (PDT) or endoluminal high-dose radiation (HDR) using brachytherapy, establishing the limitation of the lesion to the bronchial wall or to the close vicinity is essential. Here, EBUS is superior to all other imaging procedures due to the detailed analysis of the layers of the bronchial wall.

Summary and Future Perspectives

EBUS has been proven to be superior to all other imaging procedures in staging of so-called early lung cancer, lymph nodes, and infiltration of the tracheobronchial wall . Further developments such as a Doppler function, integrated sonographic endoscopes, 3D sonography, and therapeutic options using high-energy focused ultrasound (HIFU) for tissue destruction will increase the field of application. In addition, endobronchial ultrasound will play an important role in the navigation of future instruments due to the development of man–machine interfaces and robot instruments.

References

Becker HD (1995) Bronchoscopy for airway lesions. In: Wang KP, Haponik E, Mehta A (eds) Flexible Bronchoscopy. Blackwell Scient Publ, pp 136–159

Becker HD, Herth F (1999) Endobronchial Ultrasound of the airways and the mediastinum. In: Bolliger CT, Mathur PN (eds) Progress in respiratory research. Vol 30, Interventional Bronchoscopy. Karger, Basel, pp 80–93

Bülzebruck H, Bopp R, Drings P et al. (1992) New aspects in the staging of lung cancer. Cancer 70/5:1102–1110

Hürther T, Hanrath P (1990) Endobronchiale Songraphie zur Diagnostik pulmonaler und mediastinaler Tumoren. Dtsch Med Wochenschr 115:1899–1905

Lam S, Becker HD (1996) Future diagnostic procedures. In: Feins RH (ed) Thoracic endoscopy; chest surgery clinics of North America. Saunders, Philadelphia, pp 366–380

Layer G, van Kaick G (1990) Staging des nichtkleinzelligen Bronchialkarzinoms mit CT und MRT. Radiologie 30:155–163

Miyazu Y, Miyazawa T, Iwamoto Y, Kano K, Kurimoto N (2001) The role of endoscopic techniques, laser-induced fluorescence endoscopy, and endobronchial ultrasonography in choice of appropriate therapy for bronchial cancer. J Bronchol 8:10–16

Ono R, Hirano H, Egawa S, Suemasu K (1994) Bronchoscopic ultrasonography and brachytherapy in roentgenologically occult bronchogenic carcinoma. J Bronchol 1:281–287

Pothoff G, Curtius JM, Wassermann K, Junge-Hülsing M, Sechtem U, Schicha H, Hilger HH (1992) Transösophageale Echographie im Staging von Bronchialkarzinomen. Pneumologie 46:111–117

Shannon JJ, Bude RO, Orens JB et al. (1996) Endobronchial ultrasound-guided needle aspiration of mediastinal adenopathy. Am J Respir Crit Care Med 153:1424–1430

7 The White Hemithorax

C. Görg

The "white hemithorax" is primarily a radiographic finding caused by reduced radiotransparency. Although radiographic findings are of primary importance for evaluating the extent of lung opacity, occasionally the findings cannot be interpreted in such a way that the cause of the condition can be established.

Large spreading lung consolidations are homogeneous on radiographs. They may be caused by pneumonic infiltration, atelectasis, tumor growth, pleural effusion, or combinations of these. In the majority of cases, unilateral lung opacity is caused by at least reduced quantity of air in the lung, either due to compression or infiltration.

Thus, the finding of a "white hemothorax" is a sonographic challenge. In order to assess it properly, the investigator must have knowledge of the entire spectrum of thorax sonography.

Potential causes of unilateral lung opacity are listed in Table 7.1.

7.1
Predominantly Liquid Space-Occupying Mass

The cause is nearly always a fluid exudate. Sonographic evaluation is performed bearing the following features in mind:

- Echogenicity of the effusion
  - Anechoic (e.g., transudate) (Fig. 7.1)
  - Echogenic (e.g., exudate, hemothorax, pyothorax chylothorax) (Figs. 7.2–7.5)
- Evidence of fibrin strands and septa (e.g., exudate) (Fig. 7.6)
- Evidence of widespread nodular thickening of the pleura (e.g. pleural carcinomatosis, mesothelioma) (Figs. 7.1, 7.7, 7.8)
- Sonographic characterization of lung parenchyma

Table 7.1. Potential causes of unilateral lung opacity

- Predominantly liquid space-occupying mass
  - Pleural effusion
  - Pyothorax
  - Chylothorax
  - Hemothorax
- Predominantly solid space-occupying mass
  - Obstructive atelectasis
  - Lobular pneumonia
  - Tumor
  - Fibrothorax

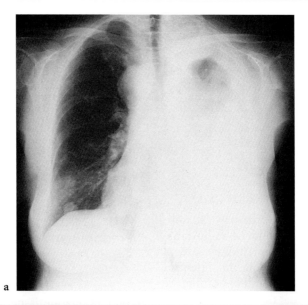

a

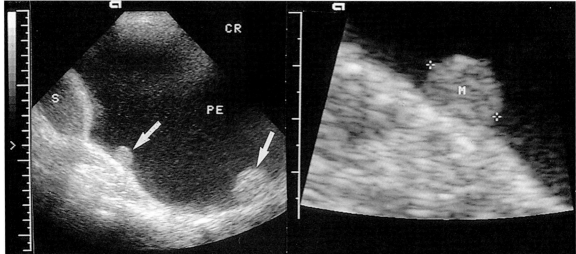

b

Fig. 7.1a, b. A 46-year-old woman with breast carcinoma. **a** Chest radiograph. Nearly complete opacity of the lung on the left side. **b** Sonography. The lateral intercostal transmission of the ultrasound beam on the left side shows a marked pleural effusion (*PE*) with small foci about 1 cm in size lying on the diaphragm and the mediastinal pleura (*arrows*). Pleural carcinomatosis was confirmed on cytology. *S*, spleen; *CR*, cranial; *M*, metastasis

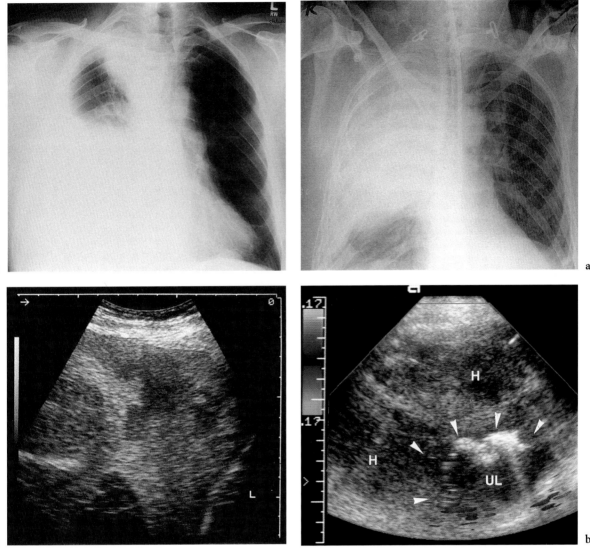

Fig. 7.2. a, b A 60-year-old man with bronchial carcinoma.
a Chest radiograph. Nearly complete lung opacity on the
right side. **b** Ultrasonography. The lateral intercostal ultrasound beam transmission on the right side shows an inhomogeneous hyperechoic structure that corresponds to respiration-dependent mobile echoes. Thoracentesis of the
effusion confirmed a hemothorax

Fig. 7.3 a, b. A 45-year-old man with sepsis and consump-
tion coagulopathy, on long-term artificial respiration.
a Chest radiograph. Almost complete opacity of the lung on
the right side. **b** Ultrasonography. The lateral intercostal
ultrasound beam transmission on the right side shows a
complex intrathoracic consolidation with no evidence of
flow phenomena on color-Doppler sonography. Aerated
lung tissue is seen in the central portion. The patient
underwent surgery and a large hematoma (*H*) in the thorax
was removed. *Arrows* indicate the upper lobes (*UL*)

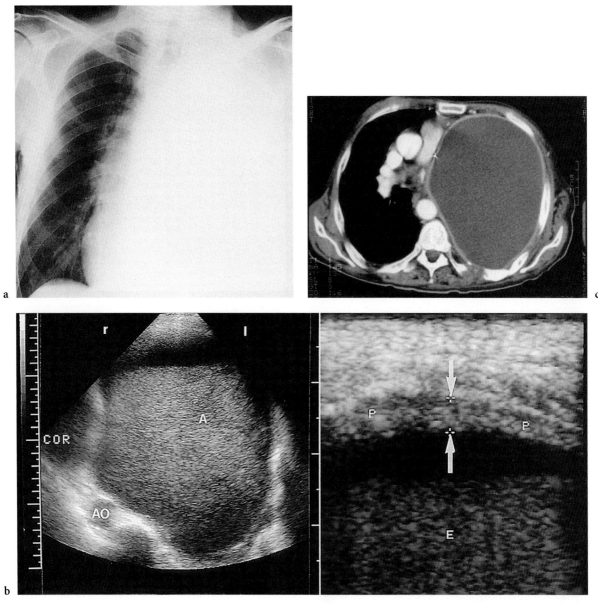

a

c

b

Fig. 7.4a–c. A 60-year-old man with high fever; bronchial carcinoma after left-sided pneumonectomy. **a** Chest radiograph. Complete opacity of the hemithorax on the left side. **b** Ultrasonography. The lateral intercostal ultrasound beam transmission on the left side shows an echogenic effusion (*A*) with sedimentation phenomena. In the vicinity of this entity, the pleura is thickened (*P*) to 5 mm (*arrows*). Diagnostic puncture produced purulent fluid, indicative of a pyothorax. *AO*, aorta; *E*, empyema; *COR*, heart. **c** Computed tomography. Homogeneous space-occupying mass with prominent walls, filling the hemithorax

Fig. 7.5a–c. A 74-year-old woman with metastatic mucus-producing ovarian carcinoma. **a** Chest radiograph. Nearly complete opacity of the lung on the right side. **b** Ultrasonography. The ventral intercostal ultrasound beam transmission on the right side shows an inhomogeneous echogenic space-occupying mass with discrete respiration-dependent, mobile echoes. Puncture produced mucinous material from a displacing, mucus-forming metastasis in the presence of ovarian carcinoma. *COR*, heart; *R*, right; *L*, left; *AO*, aorta. **c** Computed tomography. Homogeneous space-occupying mass filling the hemithorax ▶

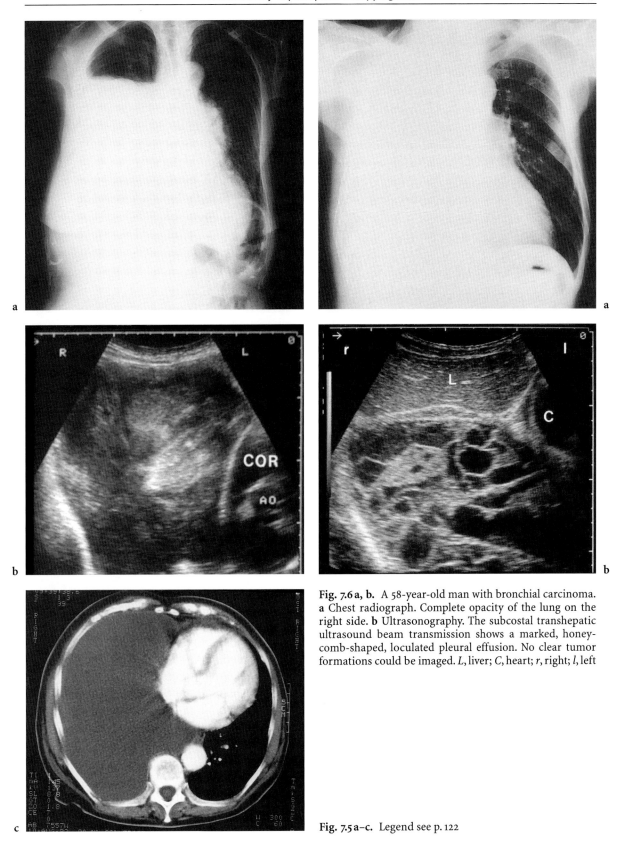

Fig. 7.6 a, b. A 58-year-old man with bronchial carcinoma. **a** Chest radiograph. Complete opacity of the lung on the right side. **b** Ultrasonography. The subcostal transhepatic ultrasound beam transmission shows a marked, honeycomb-shaped, loculated pleural effusion. No clear tumor formations could be imaged. *L*, liver; *C*, heart; *r*, right; *l*, left

Fig. 7.5 a–c. Legend see p. 122

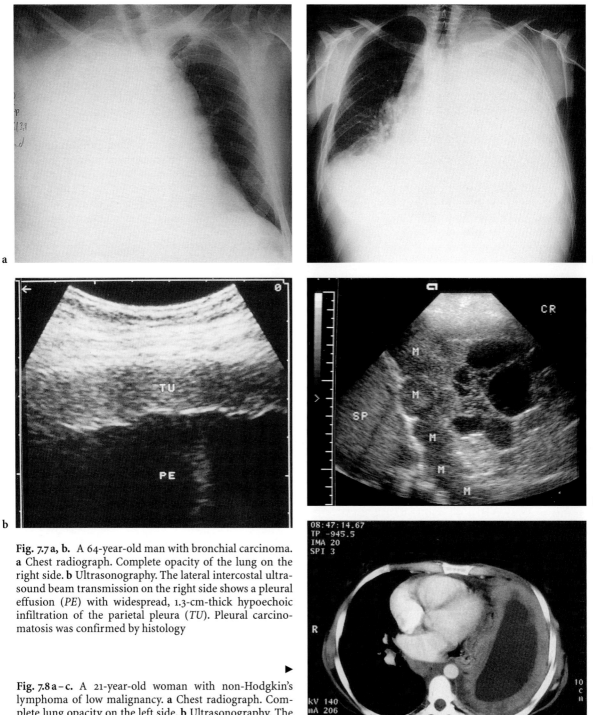

Fig. 7.7 a, b. A 64-year-old man with bronchial carcinoma. **a** Chest radiograph. Complete opacity of the lung on the right side. **b** Ultrasonography. The lateral intercostal ultrasound beam transmission on the right side shows a pleural effusion (*PE*) with widespread, 1.3-cm-thick hypoechoic infiltration of the parietal pleura (*TU*). Pleural carcinomatosis was confirmed by histology

▶

Fig. 7.8 a – c. A 21-year-old woman with non-Hodgkin's lymphoma of low malignancy. **a** Chest radiograph. Complete lung opacity on the left side. **b** Ultrasonography. The lateral intercostal ultrasound beam transmission on the left side shows a markedly loculated pleural effusion. Along the diaphragmatic pleura there are moniliform nodular tumor formations (*M*). Lymphoma of the pleura was confirmed by cytology. *CR*, cranial; *SP*, spleen. **c** Computed tomography. Widespread tumor infiltration of the pleura

7.2
Predominantly Solid Space-Occupying Mass

A solid space-occupying mass is assessed bearing the following features in mind:

- Homogeneity of the space-occupying mass (e.g., atelectasis, tumor, fibrothorax) (Figs. 7.9–7.12)
  - "Air bronchogram" (e.g., pneumonia, atelectasis) (Figs. 7.13–7.16)
  - "Fluid bronchogram" (e.g.; atelectasis) (Fig. 7.17)
  - Focal intraparenchymatous foci (e.g., metastasis, necrosis, abscess) (Figs. 7.18–7.20)
- Possible imaging of a central space-occupying mass (e.g., carcinoma, lymphoma)
- Qualitative and quantitative color-Doppler sonography of the solid space-occupying mass (Figs. 7.3, 7.9, 7.18).

With regard to the differential diagnosis of sonographic findings, the reader is referred to the preceding chapters.

In the following, the spectrum of sonographic manifestations of the white hemithorax are presented in the form of a pictorial essay.

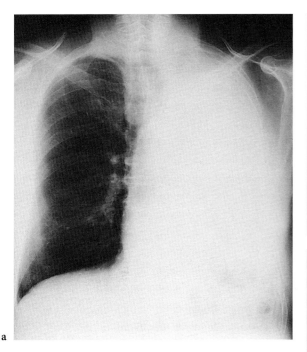

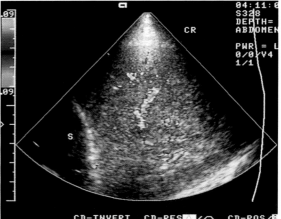

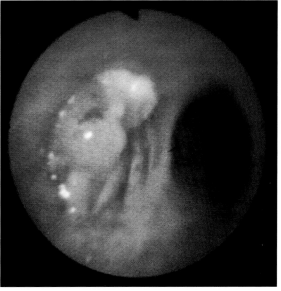

Fig. 7.9 a–c. A 68-year-old man with bronchial carcinoma. a Chest radiograph. Complete opacity of the lung on the left side. b Ultrasonography. The lateral intercostal ultrasound beam transmission on the left side shows a homogeneously hyperechoic supradiaphragmatic space-occupying mass with marked flow signals on color-Doppler sonography, corresponding to right-sided pulmonary atelectasis. *CR*, cranial; *S*, spleen. c Bronchoscopy. Complete tumor-related obstruction of the main bronchus on the left side

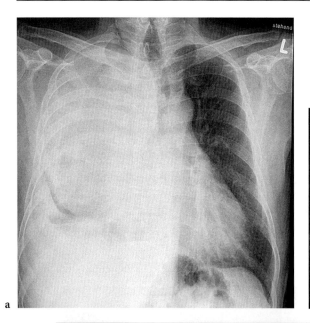

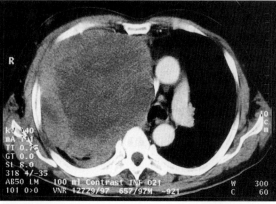

a

c

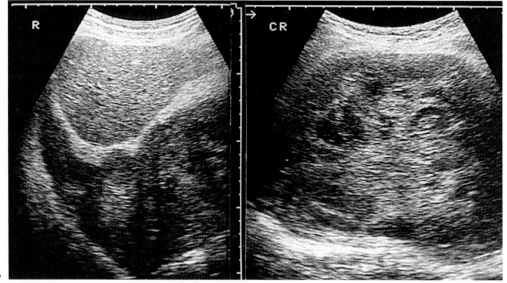

b

Fig. 7.10 a – c. A 60-year-old man with a peripheral neuro-endocrine tumor. **a** Chest radiograph. Nearly complete opacity of lung parenchyma on the side. **b** Ultrasonography. The subcostal transhepatic ultrasound beam transmission (*left image*) shows a small pleural effusion and a large solid tumor in a subdiaphragmatic location. The lateral intercostal ultrasound beam transmission on the right side (*right image*) reveals the complex tumor that nearly fills the hemithorax. *CR*, cranial. **c** Computed tomography. Large tumor filling the right hemithorax

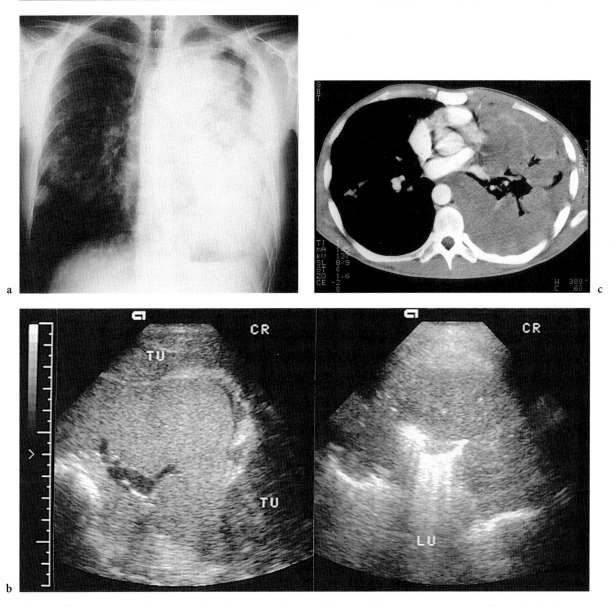

Fig. 7.11 a – c. A 34-year-old man with pulmonary blastoma. **a** Chest radiograph. Nearly complete opacity of lung parenchyma on the left side. **b** Ultrasonography. The lateral intercostal ultrasound beam transmission on the left side shows, in the caudal section (*left image*), a tumor (*TU*) that is completely infiltrating the basal diaphragmatic portions of the lung. The tumor appears to perforate the diaphragm and surrounds the spleen like a hood. In the apical portion (*right image*) the tumor walls in and invades the lung (*LU*), growing from the periphery towards the center. *CR*, cranial. **c** Computed tomography. Nearly complete tumor infiltration of the left lung

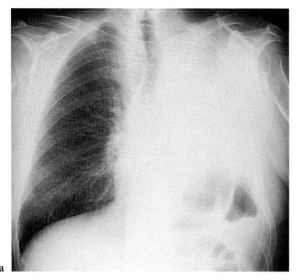

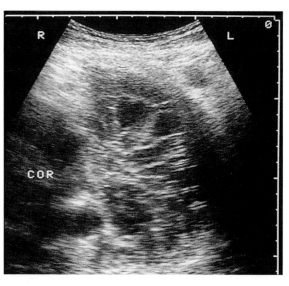

a

b

Fig. 7.12 a, b. A 65-year-old man with bronchial carcinoma, after pneumectomy. **a** Chest radiograph. Complete opacity of the lung on the left side. **b** Ultrasonography. The left-ventral intercostal ultrasound beam transmission shows an inhomogeneous, partly solid and partly cystic space-occupying mass, indicative of a fibrothorax. *R*, right; *L*, left; *COR*, heart

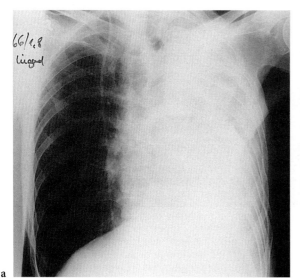

a

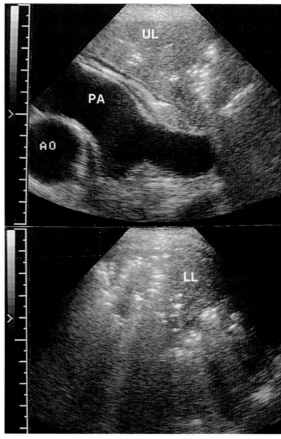

b

Fig. 7.13 a, b. A 66-year-old alcoholic, cachectic male patient with lobar pneumonia. **a** Chest radiograph. Complete opacity of the lung on the left side. **b** Ultrasonography. The left ventral intercostal ultrasound beam transmission (*upper image*) shows a nearly completely hypoechoic upper lobe with a discrete central air bronchogram. *AO*, aorta; *PA*, pulmonary artery; *UL*, upper lobe. The left-lateral intercostal ultrasound beam transmission (*lower image*) shows an invasive process with an "air bronchogram" as in pneumonia of the lower lobe (*LL*)

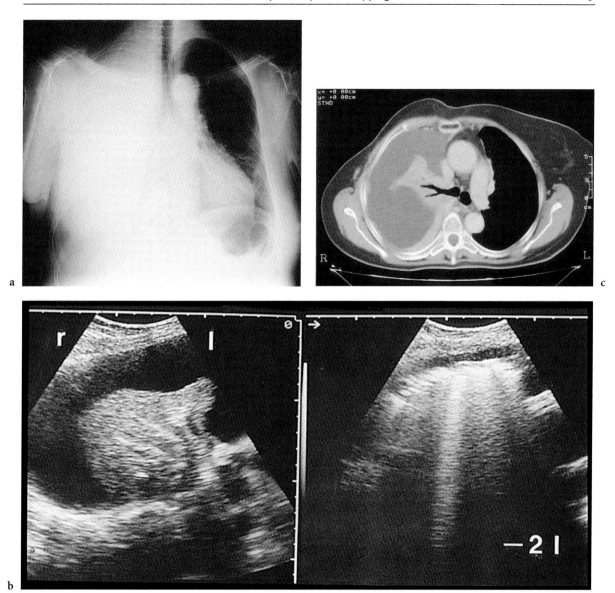

Fig. 7.14 a – c. A 61-year-old woman with breast carcinoma. **a** Chest radiograph. Complete opacity of the lung on the right side. **b** Ultrasonography. The infraclavicular right-ventral intercostal ultrasound beam transmission reveals nearly complete atelectasis of the upper lobe and a positive air bronchogram. After puncture of the effusion, the upper lobe is reventilated, as in the presence of compression atelectasis; *r*, right; *l*, left. **c** Computed tomography. Effusion with compression atelectasis of the right upper lobe

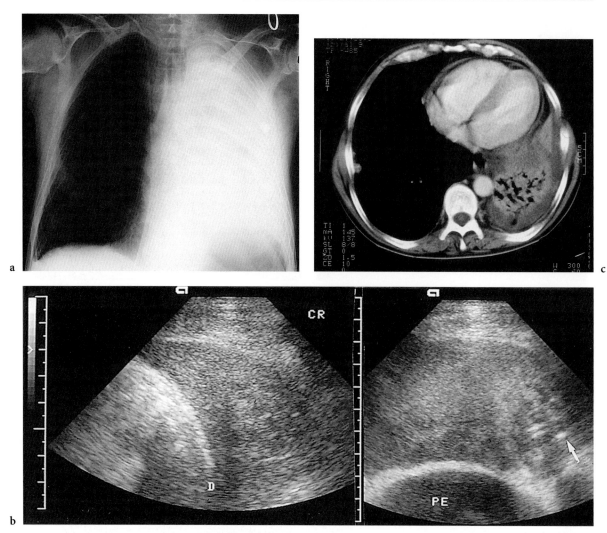

Fig. 7.15a–c. A 48-year-old alcoholic male patient with lobar pneumonia. **a** Chest radiograph. Complete opacity of the lung on the left side. **b** Ultrasonography. The left lateral intercostal ultrasound beam transmission (*left image*) and the sectional plane at right angles to it (*right image*) reveal so-called hepatization of the lung. Small air reflexes are indicative of a potential inflammatory process (*arrow*), but the appearance is nearly identical to that of atelectasis. *CR*, cranial; *D*, diaphragm; *PE*, pleural effusion formation. **c** Computed tomography. Invasive process in the left lung. Central air bronchogram

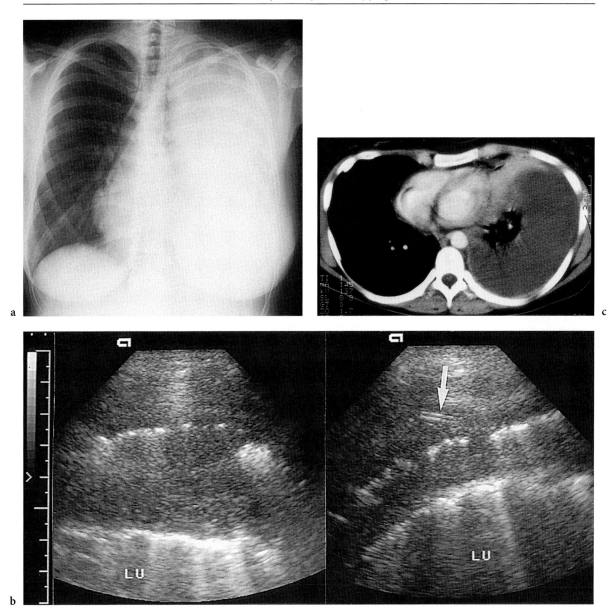

Fig. 7.16 a – c. A 30-year-old man with pneumonia. **a** Chest radiograph. Complete opacity of the lung on the left side. **b** Ultrasonography. The left-lateral intercostal ultrasound beam transmission reveals ventilated lung tissue (*LU*) in the central portion. A mantle-shaped hypoechoic transfor- mation is bordered by a narrow reflex corresponding to infiltration of the lung. An echogenic effusion identified in the pleural space is drained through a catheter (*arrow*). **c** Computed tomography. Homogeneous space-occupying mass in the left hemithorax with central aerated portions

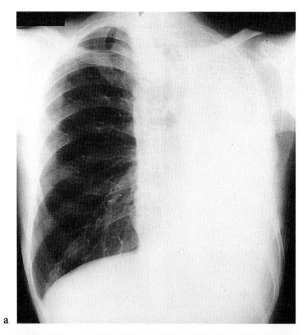

a

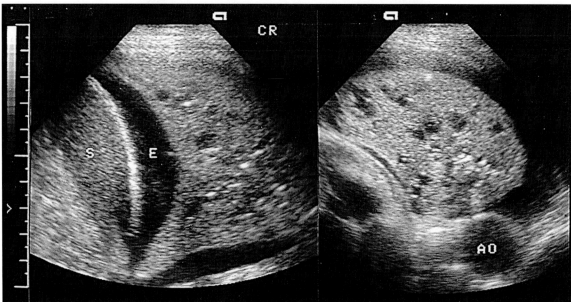

b

Fig. 7.17 a, b. A 65-year-old man with bronchial carcinoma. **a** Chest radiograph. Complete opacity of the lung on the left side. **b** Ultrasonography. The left-lateral intercostal ultrasound beam transmission (*left image*) and the sectional plane at right angles to it (*right image*) show a discrete pleural effusion and complete atelectasis of the lower lobe with multiple, dilated bronchi corresponding to a "fluid bronchogram". *S*, spleen; *E*, effusion; *AO*, aorta; *CR*, cranial

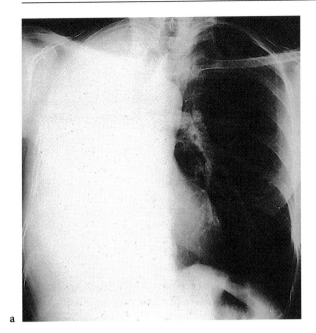

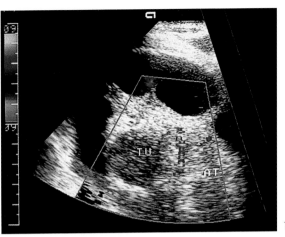

a

b

Fig. 7.18 a, b. A 64-year-old man with bronchial carcinoma. **a** Chest radiograph. Complete opacity of the lung on the right side. **b** Ultrasonography. The right-ventral intercostal ultrasound beam transmission through the upper lobe reveals a loculated pleural effusion, atelectasis of the upper lobe (*AT*) with flow signals on color-Doppler sonography, and a hypoechoic circular focus in the lung parenchyma as in metastasis (*TU*)

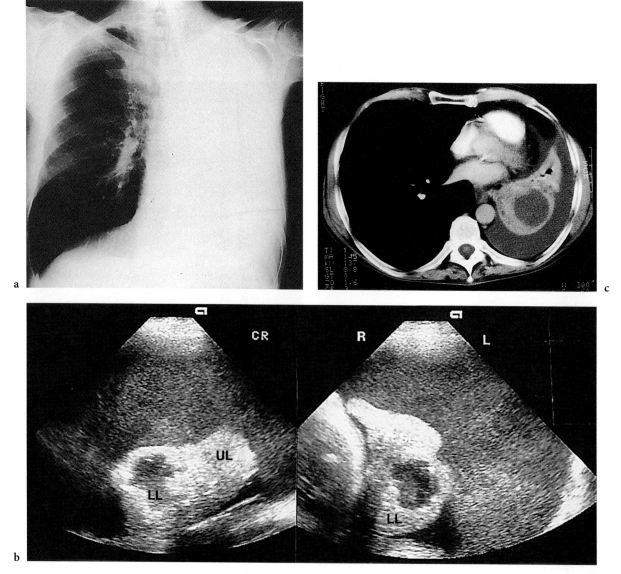

Fig. 7.19 a – c. A 63-year-old man with bronchial carcinoma. **a** Chest radiograph. Complete opacity of the lung on the left side. **b** Ultrasonography. The left-lateral intercostal ultrasound beam transmission (*left image*) and the sectional plane at right angles to it (*right image*) show a hyperechoic effusion with total atelectasis of the upper lobe (*UL*) and lower lobe (*LL*). In the central portion of the lower lobe there is a liquid space-occupying mass corresponding to colliquation (necrosis). *CR*, cranial. **c** Computed tomography. Effusion, formation of atelectasis, and central liquefaction

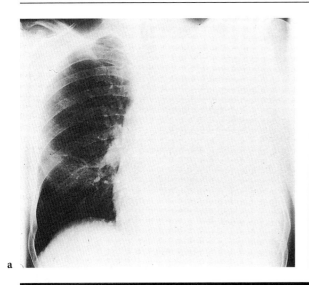

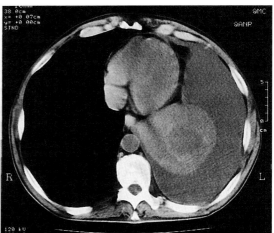

a

c

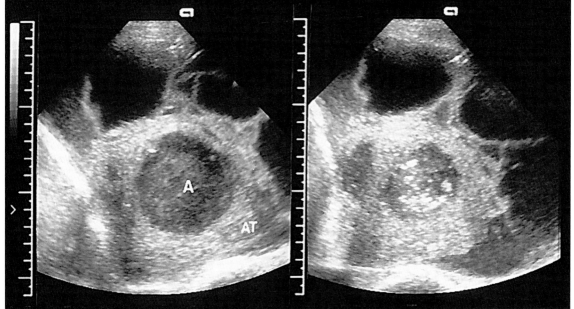

b

Fig. 7.20a–c. A 52-year-old highly febrile (temperature above 39 °C) man with bronchial carcinoma. **a** Chest radiograph. Complete opacity of the lung on the left side. **b** Ultrasonography. The left-lateral intercostal ultrasound beam transmission reveals a loculated effusion with complete atelectasis (*AT*) of the lower lobe and central liquefaction (*A*) (*left image*). The central abscess-like space-occupying mass was punctured and 120 ml of pus removed (*right image*). **c** Computed tomography. Effusion, atelectasis, and a parenchymatous space-occupying mass

8   Image Artifacts and Pitfalls

A. Schuler

The diagnostic outcome of chest ultrasonography is greatly influenced by the investigator's knowledge and careful handling of artifacts in the B-mode image (and color Doppler).

Artifacts

Artifacts are a system-immanent aspect of ultrasonography. They arise due to physical phenomena when ultrasound waves pass through the human body (see Table 8.1). Artifacts are disruptive artificial products that make it very difficult to image and evaluate the thorax, especially due to the anatomical features of this region. Artifacts can distort existing structures in terms of their size, position, form, and echogenicity; cause incorrect or incomplete imaging of their topography; or suggest the presence of structures that, in fact, do not exist. On the other hand, artifacts are indispensable and very important determinants of the diagnosis of specific diseases. The absence of certain typical artifacts (air: reverberation; bone: acoustic shadow) at the surface of the lung or in the bony thorax enables the investigator to diagnose certain diseases (lung lesion, rib lesion), as it is then possible to evaluate parenchyma, bone, and/or soft tissue. Artifacts also serve as a diagnostic criterion when they are seen at an unusual site, e.g., air with reverberation echoes in the pleural space in cases of pneumothorax.

Table 8.1. Physical phenomena of ultrasound waves

• Reflection	• Refraction
• Absorption	• Dispersion
• Diffraction	• Attenuation

Pitfalls

These are sources of error in ultrasonographic diagnosis, caused by anatomical, topographic, pathophysiological, or physical ultrasound-based misinterpretation on the part of the investigator, leading to incorrect diagnosis. Incomplete history taking, missing clinical information or examination, or insufficient knowledge of sonographic (and clinical) differential diagnosis may also be the reason for such "pitfalls." Last, but not least, every conscientious ultrasonographer must be aware of the limitations of the method so that additional diagnostic procedures can be applied efficiently, economically, and in a manner that is conducive to the patient's well-being. By so doing, several pitfalls can be avoided or resolved.

Ultrasound Physics in the Thorax

Ultrasound images are created by the transmission and passage of ultrasound waves in the human body and the registration and processing of the backscattered/received echo of the emitted ultrasound beam. In an entirely homogeneous medium, a sound wave is carried forward in a uniform fashion. It is altered at the margin between two media. The phenomena/changes that are liable to occur in this process are summarized in Table 8.1. They include the geometry of the ultrasound wave, the angle at which it strikes the reflector, the physical properties of the reflector, and its surface consistency. The magnitude of the impedance difference between two different media is represented by various factors, one of them being the intensity of the backscattered echo. Thus, on the B-mode image, it is represented by the brightness of a pixel. Human tissue contains a number of marginal sur-

faces whose anatomical origin can be determined
by characteristic ultrasound phenomena.

In contrast to the abdomen, ultrasonography of
the chest is more frequently confronted with
disturbing artifacts because of the surrounding
"echo-opposing" structures (aerated lung, bony
thorax). Therefore, the specific ultrasound phenomena in air and bony structures will be briefly
discussed in the following.

Air. This is a strong ultrasound beam reflector.
Depending on the structure of the surface, the
impedance difference and the gas volume at the
marginal surface, ultrasound waves differ in terms
of their reflex behavior:

- Large extent of absorption
- Total reflection with acoustic shadow
- Partial reflections with change of transmission
  and a narrow acoustic shadow

The most common phenomenon is that up to 99%
of the ultrasound wave is reflected at the first marginal surface between tissue and air, i.e., the "initial lung echo." Therefore, it is not possible to visualize the deeper lung parenchyma by ultrasonography. Only when the structure of the surface is
altered and in the presence of specific physical
features (e.g., the absence of air in inflammatory
or tumor-related processes, atelectasis, etc.) is it
possible to image lung parenchyma. However, in
such cases, the lung itself has several marginal surfaces (air in the bronchoalveolar space, bronchial
wall, interstitial space, vascular wall, blood). The
above-mentioned alterations in the ultrasound
wave also occur at these marginal surfaces.

Bone. In bone, there is nearly complete absorption
of ultrasound energy. As a result, the "dorsal" ultrasound wave is obliterated (no further echoes in
axial direction of the beam). When ultrasound
waves hit bone at right angles, they may cause
strong reflection and repetitive echoes of the bone
surface in deeper portions (Fig. 8.1).

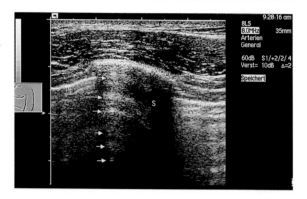

Fig. 8.1. Reflective shadowing at the clavicle (*CL*). Dorsal
acoustic shadow (*S*) due to absorption of ultrasound waves
at the surface of the clavicle. Additional reverberations
(repetitive echoes, *arrows*) at the surface of the clavicle
when the ultrasound waves hit perpendicularly. *PL*, pleural
reflex

8.1
Imaging of Marginal Surfaces
of the Pleura and the Diaphragm

The image varies, depending on the angle of incidence of ultrasound waves and the consistency
(roughness) of the surfaces. Furthermore, the
improved resolution of ultrasound probes and
continuous advancement of technology permit
differentiated imaging. At an angle of incidence of
0 to about 25°, total reflection may be expected to
occur at the marginal surface between the pleura
and the lung. Only when the surface of the pleura/
lung is thickened due to inflammation or scars
and the surface is irregular and "roughened," is it
imaged even in the presence of a steeper angle of
incidence (Mathis 1996).

Most of the diaphragm can be imaged by the trans-
abdominal approach (as a rule through the liver
from the right side and through the spleen from
the right side). Due to the high impedance difference as well as scatter phenomena, the diaphragm
is visualized as much thicker than it actually is
(Fig. 8.2). Central portions of the diaphragm
are not imaged well by the intercostal approach
because of the unfavorable angle of incidence of
the ultrasound wave. Apparent gaps might irritate
the investigator. Moreover, lateral marginal shadow
phenomena limit the assessment. Indistinct processes must be imaged in the complementary second plane.

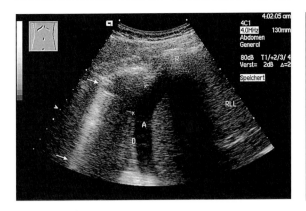

Fig. 8.2. "Diaphragmatic gap". A female patient with a primary peritoneal mesothelioma, ascites (*A*) and basal pleural pneumonia. The central portion of the diaphragm (*D*) is found to be markedly thickened. In areas close to the transducer, there seems to be a gap (*x–x*). Furthermore, a lateral marginal shadow phenomenon is seen in the diaphragm and also a comet-tail artifact in air in the cranially located lung (*arrows*). *RLL*, right lobe of liver; *R*, rib with dorsal acoustic shadow

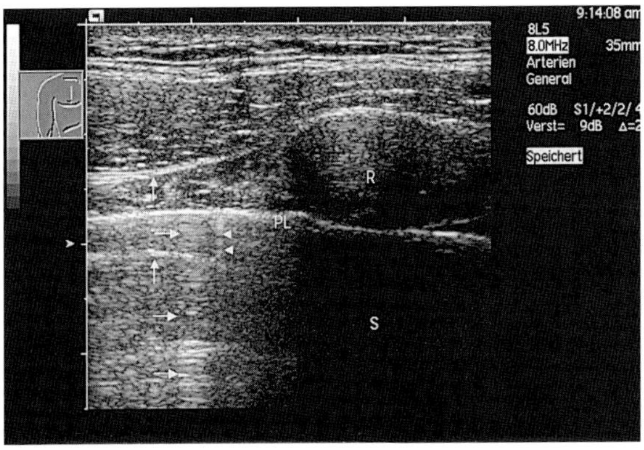

Fig. 8.3. Reverberations and comet-tail, parasternal longitudinal section from the right side. One finds reverberation artifacts (*horizontal arrows*) dorsally in the aerated lung, and a short comet-tail artifact (*arrowheads*). Furthermore, a muscle fascia of the thorax musculature is mirrored dorsally (*vertical arrows*) at the pleural reflex (*PL*). Rib (*R*) with an incomplete acoustic shadow (*S*); the pleural reflex acts as a strong reflector and is imaged here through partly cartilaginous rib with partial echo transmission

8.2
B-Mode Artifacts

Based on their mechanism of origin and physical ultrasound features, artifacts may be divided into four categories (Table 8.2; Kremkau and Taylor 1986; Schuler 1998).

Ultrasound Beam Artifacts in Thorax Sonography

Reverberations (Repetitive Echoes): Margin Between Tissue and Air, Bone Fracture Fissures

They arise due to nearly complete reflection of the emitted ultrasound wave at the marginal surface between tissue and air (initial lung echo). This marginal surface acts as a strong reflector. It reflects the striking ultrasound wave back to the

Table 8.2. Classification of artifacts

- Ultrasound beam artifacts
- Ultrasound enhancement artifacts
- Ultrasound resolution artifacts
- Other artifacts

transducer membrane, where the wave is re-reflected and re-emitted, hits the marginal surface again, etc. Depending on the duration, the marginal surface reflex is imaged dorsally, in axial direction of the ultrasound wave. Deeper reflectors are weaker and are imaged darker (Figs. 8.2, 8.3). The artifact caused by insufficient probe-to-specimen contact (see Fig. 8.10), e.g., when a linear ultrasound probe is used on the surface of the thorax, actually is a reverberation artifact (at the transducer membrane).

A narrow fissure in a rib fracture might become noticeable because of a reverberation artifact (so-called chimney phenomenon) (Dubs-Kunz 1992). The fracture end of the rib serves as a strong reflector in this setting (see Figs. 2.13, 2.14).

Mirror Artifacts: Liver Parenchyma in the Diaphragm, Vessels at the "Pleura"

These are caused by incidence-angle-dependent reflection of the ultrasound wave at a strong reflector (e.g., the diaphragm), oblique deflection in tissue, repeated reflection on a reflector, backscatter to the first reflector, and back-reflection to the ultrasound probe. This is imaged as a structure not primarily in the axial direction of the ultra-

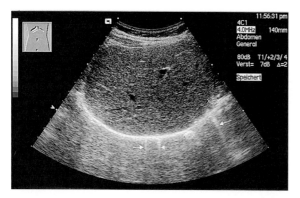

Fig. 8.4. Mirror artifact. Subcostal oblique section from the right side. "Classical" mirror artifact of the liver at the diaphragm. Portions lying at a distance from the transducer and the diaphragm, i.e., cranially by the subcostal approach, are not "lung parenchyma" but liver parenchyma reflected at the strong reflector, namely the diaphragm. A hemangioma (x–x) lying immediately subdiaphragmal in the original image is more clearly seen in the mirror image (x–x) and is displaced centrally to the mid portion of the image. In some cases, the mirror image might reveal structures outside the main beam that cannot be imaged (multiple beam artifacts) and cause considerable confusion. Additional comet-tail artifacts (*arrows*) in air

sound beam, within a region axial-distal to the actual reflector. This causes the classical mirror artifact phenomena of the liver at the diaphragm (Fig. 8.4), but also of the subclavian artery at the initial lung reflex. This artifact phenomenon exists not only in B-mode sonography, but also in color Doppler and the Doppler frequency spectrum (Fig. 8.5). As a rule, the multiple backscattered echoes of mirror images are more hypoechoic and somewhat more blurred or distorted as a result of previous weakening of the ultrasound beam when it passes through tissue.

Arcuate Artifacts: Rib Reflex in Pleural Effusion

Arcuate artifacts may arise due to displacement of a reflex at a strong reflector in the lateral ultrasound beam or side lobe into the center of the main beam. Characteristically, in sector transducers and upwardly oriented curved arrays, one finds upwardly open circular arches. In linear probes, one finds a hyperbola. Thus, a reflection in a bony portion of the thorax could mimic a septation in a pleural effusion (Fig. 8.6). This problem can be resolved by altering the echo angle or the echo plane.

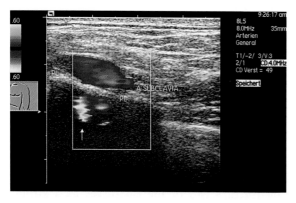

Fig. 8.5. Mirror artifact on color Doppler. The subclavian artery (*A. SUBCLAVIA*) is reflected at the pleura (*PL*). A vessel (*arrow*) lying dorsal to the pleura is seen on the mirror image; the vessel, however, does not really exist

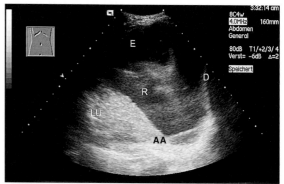

Fig. 8.6. Arcuate artifact in the pleural effusion. A female patient with pulmonary and pleural metastatic breast carcinoma. A strong reflector (bony thorax) lying outside the main beam is visualized as a circular arch (*AA*, arcuate artifact), discretely opening upward. Distally, it may mimic septation of the pleural effusion (*E*). The internal echoes (*R*) are not corpuscular portions of the effusion but noise artifacts ("speckles"). *D*, diaphragm; *LU*, lung atelectasis in the presence of pleural effusion

Scatter Lens Artifact/Shortening Phenomenon: Distortion of the Lung Surface Dorsal to Rib Cartilage

This artifact phenomenon is a result of the different transmission rates of ultrasound waves in rib cartilage (faster) than in the adjacent soft tissue of the chest wall. This may mimic a pseudolesion at the marginal surface of air/lung, because there is an apparent protrusion of contours in the direction of the ultrasound probe (Fig. 8.7). This artifact is simple to detect and plays a rather important role in abdominal diagnosis of the liver (apparent space-occupying mass on the surface of the liver) dorsal to rib cartilage (Bönhof and Linhart 1985).

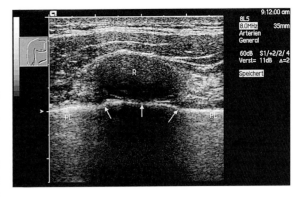

Fig. 8.7. Scatter lens artifact. The pleura (*PL*) dorsal to the rib cartilage (*R*) is shifted ventrally towards the transducer (*arrows*) as a result of various ultrasound beam rates in cartilage and soft tissue of the chest wall

Marginal Shadows: Diffraction/Refraction at Strong Reflectors ("Diaphragmatic Gap")

This artifact occurs when the ultrasound beam hits a surface obliquely. It is the result of diffraction and refraction phenomena at strong reflectors (e.g., the diaphragm; see Fig. 8.2). The artifact is detected by the fact that it disappears when the echo plane or the echo angle is changed.

Artifacts Caused by Alterations in Echo Enhancement

Acoustic Shadow/Echo Obliteration: Formation of Plaque on All Bony Structures of the Thorax

This certainly is one of the most common artifact phenomena in the thorax and greatly hinders the assessment of structures lying dorsal to such strong reflectors. Due to strong absorption, dorsal bone structures (ribs, scapula, clavicle, sternum, vertebral column) are nearly completely obliterated and practically all information is lost (see Fig. 8.1). However, interruptions of the otherwise regular acoustic shadow in the bony thorax (bone contour, bone surface, joints) may be very helpful for diagnosis, as pathological changes will be present in such cases (fracture, bone tumor, joint effusion, joint empyema). Acoustic shadows in the pleura are also signs of pathological alterations, e.g., of plaque in the presence of asbestosis or calcification during the healing of pleural lung lesions or lung lesions close to the pleura (pneumonia, tuberculosis) or in lymph nodes.

Echo Enhancement: Distal to Hypoechoic Structures (Pleural Effusion, Cyst, Vessel, Hypoechoic Space-Occupying Mass)

This phenomenon of "brighter," more hyperechoic areas distal to the above-mentioned structures is not due to echo enhancement but due to lesser weakening of ultrasound waves in the more hypoechoic portions closer to the probe. This causes distal parts to appear brighter (more hyperechoic and stronger echoes) than the surrounding areas, which have uniformly weakened echoes. In the thorax, this is found in the presence of large quantities of fluid in the pleural space or hypoechoic peripheral pulmonary processes (Figs. 8.8, 8.9).

Echo Resolution Artifacts

Noise: In Fluid-Filled Structures

At the surface of anechoic areas, one finds diffuse "noise" caused by interference from returning echoes at different marginal surfaces, such as those caused by "background noise," depending on general enhancement (this is also true for Doppler sonography). Here caution is advised, as apparently internal structures that in fact do not exist might be mimicked (e.g., in the pleural effusion; Figs. 8.6, 8.8). Marginal surfaces are frequently blurred.

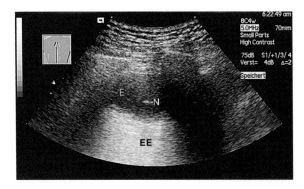

Fig. 8.8. Echo enhancement. Dorsal to a small, not entirely anechoic pleural effusion (*E*) there is marked "echo enhancement" (*EE*). This actually is reduced weakening of the echo, as the spread of the ultrasound beam in the pleural effusion is altered in comparison with adjacent tissue. Also note the nonanechoic effusion close to the chest wall. The reflexes are noise artifacts. Furthermore, an echodense small bright linear reflex (*N*) is seen, the tip of the puncture needle introduced under sonographic guidance

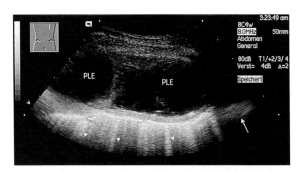

Fig. 8.9. Comet-tail and probe-to-specimen artifact. Dorsal to a septate pleural effusion in the presence of breast carcinoma one finds numerous comet-tail artifacts (*arrowheads*) arising in the air at the margin between the visceral pleura and the lung. Furthermore, given insufficient contact between the ultrasound probe and the chest wall, a shadow with an artifact reflex (*arrow*), although not like a classical ring-down artifact. Dorsal to the pleural effusion, there is marked echo enhancement. *PLE*, pleural effusion

Slice Thickness Artifact: At Reflectors with a Strong Impedance Difference (Pleura, Diaphragm)

This common and irritating artifact also belongs to the category of resolution artifacts. When the ultrasound beam hits strong reflectors obliquely and in the presence of a high impedance difference, the marginal layer is much thicker, (partly) blurred, and distorted. This phenomenon might mimic pleural and diaphragmatic lesions or thickening (see Fig. 8.2), but also thrombosis or sediments in vessels.

Other Artifacts

Comet-Tail (Resonance Artifact): In Aerated Structures

At the margin of the lung surface and air one frequently finds small comet-tail artifacts (see Figs. 8.2–8.4, 8.9). They are seen as bright, narrow strips of strong dorsal reflectors and their origin is controversially discussed. One explanation is reverberations (repetitive echoes) between two very closely located reflectors and resonance phenomena (vibrations) with a strong echo response. In addition to air or other gas bubbles, a common site of origin is metal foreign bodies.

Artifacts Caused by Foreign Bodies: Needle Tip, Drainage

Iatrogenic or accidental foreign bodies introduced into the body cause artifact phenomena. As a result, projectiles, fragments of glass or wood, or other substances might be imaged in the chest wall and in soft tissue. This is significant when such artifacts are visualized during sonography-guided diagnostic or therapeutic measures. Small pulmonary consolidations close to the pleura, pleural effusions a few millimeters in size, or pleural empyema can be punctured or drained under real-time sonographic guidance. Space-occupying masses in the soft tissue of the thorax or rib cage should also be punctured under sonographic guidance. Detection of the needle reflex in aerated structures might be difficult. Here, real-time control through subtle movement of the needle tip under simultaneous sonographic imaging is useful (Fig. 8.8; Blank 1994).

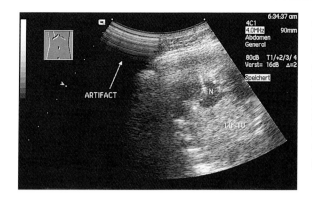

Fig. 8.10. Ring-down (probe-to-specimen artifact). Patient with a peripheral bronchial carcinoma in a ventral location on the right side. A probe-to-specimen artifact (*arrow*) is caused by insufficient contact between the transducer and the chest wall. A simultaneous fine-needle puncture performed for histological verification of the diagnosis shows the needle artifact (*N*) in the tumor (*LU-TU*)

Ring-Down Artifact:
Insufficient Probe-to-Specimen Contact

If the geometric configuration of the probe is unfavorable in relation to the investigated region (for instance a linear probe in a curved chest wall), this artifact can easily be detected by characteristic repetitive echoes (arising between the ultrasound crystal and the transducer membrane) (Fig. 8.10).

8.3
Color Doppler Artifacts and Pitfalls in the Thorax

The basic principles and settings of the various Doppler modalities will not be presented in this chapter. They have been discussed in detail elsewhere (Wild 1996).

Pulse Repetition Frequency, Overall Enhancement, Filter, Background Noise

Insufficient or incorrect setting of the overall enhancement of color Doppler either leads to incorrect imaging of actual blood flow (excessively low gain) or "over-radiation" due to numerous color pixels that do not represent blood flow but only background noise (poor signal-to-noise ratio).

A low pulse repetition frequency (PRF) should be selected for small vessels with low flow rates so that flow signals are not "overlooked." When large arteries are visualized (mediastinum, suprasternal, parasternal), it may be necessary to increase the PRF or reduce overall enhancement. The same is true for spectral Doppler. Selection of the wall filter should also be controlled, so that slow flow signals or signals of low intensity are not "filtered away."

Directional Artifact

The directional artifact is not actually an artifact phenomenon but evidence of directionally encoded visualization of blood flow on color Doppler (Fig. 8.11). Thus, in a vessel with blood flow in the opposite direction of the ultrasound probe (for instance, when the vessel has a curved flow), the colors red and blue will be present in one and the same vessel. The actual change in the direction of blood flow is seen at the margin of the two colors; this area will be black (corresponding to null flow; see color scale).

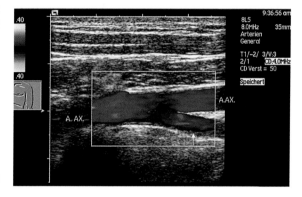

Fig. 8.11. Directional artifact (color Doppler). The axillary artery (infraclavicular) (*A. AX.*) with a branch for the musculature/chest wall. Blood flowing towards the ultrasound probe is coded red; blood flowing away from the probe is coded blue (see color scale). The branching artery (*arrow*) is blue, the change of color from red to blue occurs via black. Thus, here (at a 90° Doppler angle to the ultrasound probe), there is no blood flow relative to the ultrasound probe

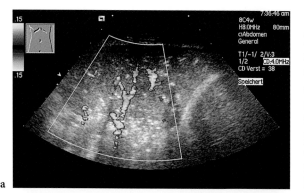

a

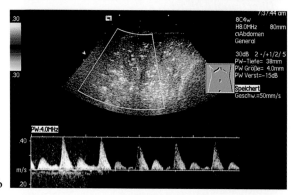

b

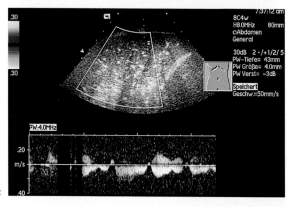

c

Aliasing

In contrast to directional artifacts, aliasing is marked by a change of color through the bright color zones. This phenomenon is expressed as a colorful mosaic in the transition zone between two colors and will be seen at higher flow rates than the selected PRF (Fig. 8.12 a). In spectral Doppler, portions of higher frequency appear as being "cut off" at the lower or upper margin of the Doppler frequency spectrum. Aliasing shows, for instance, higher-grade stenosis and disturbance of flow within vessels (Fig. 8.13). Increasing the PRF of color and spectral Doppler (up to the Nyquist limit) will help at least to reduce aliasing. It might also be possible to clearly determine the direction of flow (Fig. 8.12 b, c).

Motion Artifacts

Mechanical movement of tissue against the ultrasound probe (breathing, musculature, cardiac and vascular pulsation, etc.) causes an apparent "frequency shift," which creates a signal in color Doppler as well. This disturbs, in particular, the assessment of structures close to the heart and

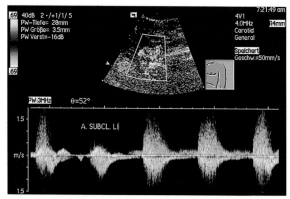

Fig. 8.12. a Aliasing on color Doppler in a pulmonary vessel in the presence of pneumonia. Given a low pulse repetition frequency in color Doppler (color scale, here 15 cm/s), color alone does not permit the investigator to conclusively establish the direction of flow. The change of color in the vessel is achieved via brighter colors. Thus, the mean flow rate in this vessel is more than 15 cm/s. **b** Pulmonary artery. Only when pulse repetition frequency is increased to 30 cm/s is it possible to clearly distinguish pulmonary vessels. On red color coding, color Doppler shows an afferent artery. On spectral Doppler, the corresponding Doppler frequency spectrum, suggesting four-phase flow. **c** Pulmonary vein. Blue color coding shows centrally aligned blood flow. Spectral Doppler shows the venous flow signal

Fig. 8.13. Stenosis of the subclavian artery. In spite of high pulse repetition frequency (maximum 69 cm/s), there is markedly faster flow within the vessel, which is imaged by the bright color pixels in the vessel. Furthermore, the vessel itself is poorly delineated; color pixels are also seen outside of it. This is also known as a vibration artifact and is caused by tissue vibration secondary to stenosis and due to concomitant pulsations that cannot be reliably distinguished from the vessel in terms of space. Spectral Doppler shows flow maxima of about 1.5 m/s and retrograde flow (below the null line), as well as pathological, non-triphasic flow in this extremity artery

vessels due to persistent superimposition, and is a limitation of the method, e.g., in the detection of low blood flow in such areas. Various "artifact suppression" modalities proposed by manufacturers of ultrasound devices have achieved some improvement in this regard. Even in the presence of stenosis, movement of tissue due to concomitant motion (vibrations) on color Doppler might represent apparent flow signals outside the vessel (Fig. 8.13).

Unfavorable Angles

An angle of >60–90° may lead to incorrect Doppler measurements or incorrect imaging of blood flow (color Doppler and spectral Doppler). In such cases, the modality of power Doppler would at least help to image vessels in the thorax/lung (Yang 1996). In this setting, a largely angle-independent, directionally non-encoded, more sensitive documentation of blood flow is achieved by the visualization of amplitude (not frequency shift) of the backscattering echo.

Summary

On the one hand, artifacts are disturbing synthetic products which render visualization and assessment especially difficult in the chest because of the special anatomical features of this region. On the other hand, the absence of typical artifacts at the surface of the lung or the bony thorax makes it possible to diagnose certain diseases in the first place (subpleural lung lesion, rib fracture), as it allows assessment of parenchyma or bone. Finally, artifacts also serve as a diagnostic criterion, e.g., air with reverberation echoes in the pleural space in the presence of pneumothorax.

References

Blank W (1994) Sonographisch gesteuerte Punktionen und Drainagen. In: Braun B, Günther RW, Schwerk WB (Hrsg) Ultraschalldiagnostik Lehrbuch und Atlas. ecomed, Landsberg. Bd III/11.1, S 20 f

Bönhof JA, Bönhof B, Linhart P (1984) Acoustic dispersing lenses cause artifactual discontinuities in B-mode ultrasonograms. J Ultrasound Med 3:5–7

Bönhof JA, Linhart P (1985) A pseudolesion of the liver caused by rib cartilage in B-mode ultrasonography. J Ultrasound Med 4:135–137

Dubs-Kunz B (1992) Sonographische Diagnostik von Rippenfrakturen. In: Anderegg A, Despland P, Henner H (Hrsg) Ultraschalldiagnostik 91. Springer, Berlin Heidelberg New York Tokyo, S 286–273

Kremkau FW, Taylor KJW (1986) Artifacts in Ultrasound Imaging. J Ultrasound Med 5:227–237

Mathis, G (1996) Lungen- und Pleurasonographie. 2. Aufl., Springer, Berlin Heidelberg New York Tokyo, S 110

Reading CC, Charboneau JW, Allison JW, Cooperberg PL (1990) Color and spectral doppler mirror-image artifact of the subclavian artery. Radiology 174:41–42

Schuler A (1998) Untersuchungstechnik und Artefakte. In: Braun B, Günter RW, Schwerk WB (Hrsg) Ultraschalldiagnostik Lehrbuch und Atlas, Bd I. ecomed, Landsberg, S 1–42

Wild K (1996) Periphere Gefäße. In: Braun B (Hrsg.) Ultraschalldiagnostik Lehrbuch und Atlas, ecomed Landsberg, S 10–13

Yang PC (1996) Color doppler ultrasound of pulmonary consolidation. European J Ultrasound 3:169–178

9   Interventional Chest Sonography

W. Blank

The etiology of many diseases in chest organs can be determined by a combined evaluation of the patient's history, clinical findings, and diagnostic imaging procedures. A definitive evaluation, however, often requires additional biochemical, microbiological, cytological, or histological expert assessment. The material needed for such investigations can be obtained by targeted puncture. Given the appropriate indication, the puncture may be followed by interventional therapeutic measures (Table 9.1).

General Indications

In addition to the frequently use of puncture in the presence of effusion, space-occupying masses accessible to sonographic investigation, located in the chest wall, pleura, lung or anterior mediastinum, are important indications. (Table 9.2) (Braun 1983; Börner 1986; Weiss and Weiss 1994; Pedersen et al. 1986).

Because of the potential risk of complications, the indication for the procedure should be established with care. Punctures should only be performed when they are expected to have therapeutic consequences (e.g., radiation therapy, chemotherapy). A potentially malignant peripheral tumor in an operable patient should not be punctured, but rather immediately resected (Blank 1994; Beckh and Bölcskei 1997).

Contraindications

Severe blood coagulation disorders (Quick value < 50%, thrombocytes < 60,000) are absolute contraindications. Bullous pulmonary emphysema and pulmonary hypertension are relative contraindications. When respiratory function is severely

Table 9.1. Interventional measures in the thorax: various procedures

- Percutaneous access
  Sonography
  Radiographs (fluoroscopy, CT)
- Endoluminal access
  Bronchoscopy
  Endoluminal sonography
- Surgical (mediastinoscopy, thoracoscopy, surgical exposure)

Table 9.2. Interventions in the thorax: indications

- Space-occupying mass in the thorax wall (tumors, abscesses, hematomas, changes in the skeleton)
- Space-occupying masses in the pleura
- Pleural effusion and pleural empyema (very small quantities, loculated effusions)
- Peripheral lung consolidations (lung tumor, pneumonia, lung abscess)
- Mediastinal processes (anterior mediastinum)

restricted or blood gas values are poor, a puncture should only be performed when the patient's condition is expected to be improved by the therapeutic intervention. High-risk puncture sites should be avoided (Yang et al. 1992; Mathis 1999a).

9.1
Ultrasound- or Computed Tomography-Guided Puncture

In several diseases of the lung and mediastinum, computed tomography provides the best overview. However, it should be used as an interventional measure only when the target and pathway of puncture cannot be reliably assessed with sonography (Blank 1994; Mathis 1997a).

The *advantages* of ultrasound-guided puncture are manifold: fast availability, low complication rate, the absence of radiation, and low costs. In contrast to computed tomography-guided puncture, the puncture can be carefully observed during ultrasonography. The investigator is free to use the pathway he desires in terms of direction; the ventilated lung is protected (low rate of pneumothorax). Vessels are detected with color Doppler sonography (CDS) (upper thorax aperture, parasternal). Active vascularized portions of tumor can be punctured in a targeted fashion. Atelectatic or pneumonic parts of peripheral lung consolidations can be demarcated with CDS (Wang et al. 1995; Yang 1996).

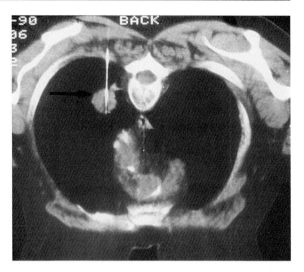

Fig. 9.2. Computed tomography-assisted puncture of a round lung center (*arrow*) which cannot be depicted by sonography, with a cutting biopsy needle (Tru-Cut 0.9 mm). The needle can be seen in longitudinal section. Histology: small-cell bronchial carcinoma

However, ultrasound-guided percutaneous puncture also has its *limitations*. If the space-occupying mass cannot be seen percutaneously on sonography, other endoluminal procedures (bronchoscopy, endoluminal sonography) may be used or a computer-assisted puncture performed (Figs. 9.1, 9.2) (Klose 1996, Mikloweit et al. 1991).

In principle, the interventional procedure that is the fastest means of arriving at the diagnosis and is the least stressful for the patient should be used.

> **In US you see what you do, in CT you see what you have done.** (Heilo 1996)

9.2
Apparatus, Instruments, and Puncture Technique

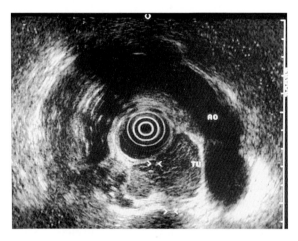

Fig. 9.1. Transesophageal mediastinal sonography (radial probe, 7.5 MHz). Hypoechoic tumor formation (*TU*) in the posterior mediastinum, located between the aortic arch and the spinal column. A fine-needle puncture has been carried out using aspiration technique. The needle can only be seen in outline between the *arrows*. The needle can be guided better with a longitudinal probe. Cytology: highly malign non-Hodgkin lymphoma. *AO*, aorta

In lesions of the chest wall, the investigator should use high-frequency linear probes. Lesions in the pleural space and lung should be investigated with sector-like probes equipped with a narrow covering. For endosonography-guided puncture, special intraluminal probes with biopsy canals are available (Kelbel et al. 1996).

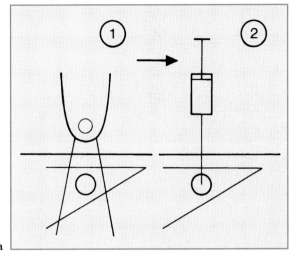

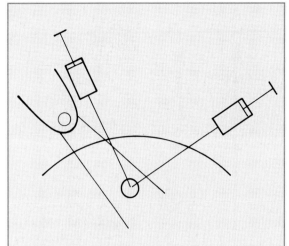

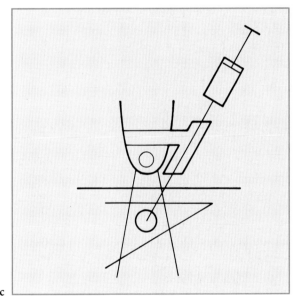

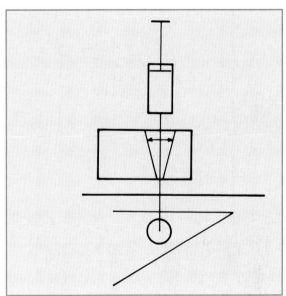

Fig. 9.3 a–d. Various puncture methods. **a** Free puncture. Free-hand puncture after sonographic location. Inexpensive, two-step method (no visual surveillance of the target area during the puncture). Very suitable for small processes located on the surface. **b** Puncture under sonographic observation. Low cost, puncture route variable, so punctures are possible from various areas, needle very visible, difficult with small processes located on the surface. Sterile gloves should be used for therapeutic operations. **c** Guided puncture. Sector/curved-array scanner with attachment. Relatively cheap, needle is easily visible, but poor view at close range, puncture route prescribed, but can be super-imposed electronically, disinfection of the attachment necessary. Not advisable on the thorax. **d** Puncture ultrasound probe. Expensive, puncture route not very variable, limited imaging through the perforation region, needle not easily visible, good view at close range. Seldom necessary for chest punctures

The puncture needle can be steered in many ways (Fig. 9.3). A simple and economical method is so-called *free puncture*. Ninety per cent of interventions are performed by the free-hand technique under sonographic visual control.

Puncture Needles

A distinction is made between fine (diameter, <1 mm) and gross needles (diameter, >1 mm) (Fig. 9.4). The rate of complications increases with the thickness of the needle and the duration of the

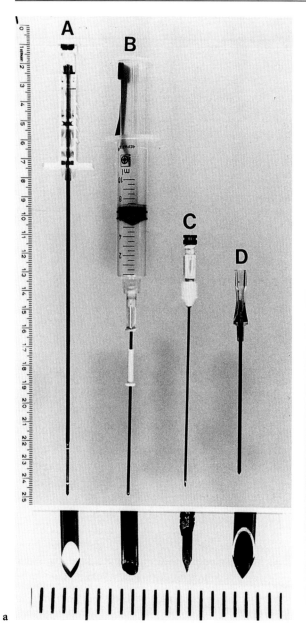

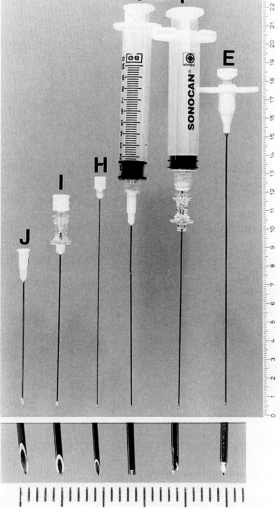

a

b

Fig. 9.4a, b. Puncture needles. **a** Coarse needles. *A*, Tru-Cut needle, diameter 1.4–2 mm; *B*, Menghini needle, diameter 1.6 mm; *C*, bone punch needle (Angiomed); *D*, aspiration needle for viscose liquids, diameter 2.0 mm. **b** Fine needles. *E*, Vaku-Cut needle based on Köhler (Angiomed). When the puncture destination has been reached, the stiletto is withdrawn three-quarters of its length to create a partial vacuum. Diameter 0.8–1.2 mm. *F*, Sonocan biopsy needle (Braun, Melsungen), diameter 0.8–1.4 mm, length 100–160 mm. Puncture technique as for the Otto needle, but without any rotating movement. *G*, cutting biopsy needle based on Otto with mandrin (Angiomed), diameter 0.8–1.2 mm, length, 100–200 mm. *H*, Chiba needle with mandrin, diameter 0.6–0.9 mm. *I*, lumbar puncture cannula with mandrin, diameter 0.9 mm. *J*, puncture cannula with no mandrin, diameter 0.7 mm

procedure. The *ideal puncture needle* should fulfill the following criteria: It should be as thin as possible, sufficiently stiff to maintain the direction of puncture, cut sharply, be such that it can be advanced forward fast, and be able to obtain sufficient material for investigation (Weiss and Düntsch 1996; Westkott 1988).

Fine Needles

For *aspiration cytology*, fine needles with a diameter of 0.6–0.8 mm are sufficient. They are available with and without a mandrel and have no cutting tip (economical injection needles, spinal puncture needles and Chiba needles). Mandrels are useful in this setting.

Puncture Technique. Once the puncture target is reached, the puncture is performed in a fan-like fashion under suction (Fig. 9.5). During forward and backward movement, cells are peeled off and aspirated into the tube. No suction should be applied during backward movement, so that material is not sucked into the syringe and dissemination of tumor tissue into the puncture canal is avoided.

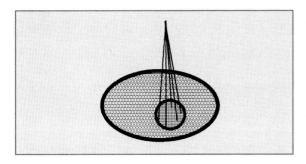

Fig. 9.5. Fine-needle aspiration puncture. Fan-shaped puncture technique

Table 9.3. Sources of error in aspiration cytology

- Poor puncture technique
- Insufficient, or no, material for evaluation (in some cases re-puncture)
- Aspiration of blood
- Incorrect smear or fixation technique
- Limited experience in cytology

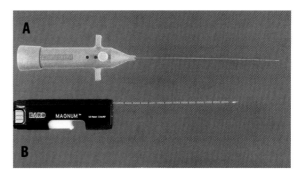

Fig. 9.6. Puncture pistols. The required depth of injection (measured sonographically) can be pre-set. *A,* Auto-Vac puncture, disposable set (Angiomed). *B,* reusable pistol (Barth) with insertable Tru-Cut needles. The Tru-Cut needle contains a biopsy chamber. Advantage: the cut cylinder of tissue cannot be lost when the needle is withdrawn. Disadvantage: short tissue cylinder

The material obtained by this procedure usually only allows a cytological investigation that is able to distinguish between malignant and benign disease; it does not permit the investigator to determine the type of malignant lesion (e.g., lymphomas). Sources of error in aspiration cytology are numerous (Table 9.3) (Blank 1994).

Cutting Biopsy Needles. Tissue cylinders for histological assessment can be obtained with these needles. One-hand needles are useful, as one investigator performs the sonographic investigation and the puncture. Puncture guns are particularly suitable in the thorax, as the puncture procedure is fast, does not require the investigator to avoid the lung, and very representative puncture cylinders can be punched out from soft tissue (Fig. 9.6). Disadvantages are the cumbersome procedure and the absence of the sensation of performing a puncture (Mathis 1997b).

Gross Needles

Gross needles (1.2–2 mm) are needed for histological differentiation, especially in benign processes of the chest wall, pleural disease, or even interstitial lung lesions (Gleeson et al. 1990; Ikezoe et al. 1990).

Drainage Catheter

The diameter of the selected catheter depends on the viscosity of the liquid formation. In principle, the drainage may be performed using the trocar or the Seldinger technique. The *trocar technique* is commonly used in the thorax (Fig. 9.7). Both drainage techniques are preceded by a diagnostic fine needle puncture.

Checking the Position of the Needle and the Catheter

Correct *placement of the needle* is not demonstrated by sonography alone. Moreover, the "sensation of puncture" usually changes when the target of puncture is reached. Optical visualization of the needle depends on the angle of the needle and the ultrasound beam. Ideally, when a needle is introduced at the level of the transducer, the needle shaft is seen as an echogenic double reflex. However, in deeper lesions, only the tip of the needle is seen as a bright double reflex (Fig. 9.8). In tissue with high echodensity it may be difficult to localize the needle. Here, it is useful to move the needle or the mandrel backwards and forwards and even employ brief suction. Color Doppler sonography will show the needle as a colored line (Fig. 9.9). When a gun is used, the incision canal (air) is visible even several seconds after the puncture. The *drainage catheter* is typically visualized as a bright double contour. On color-Doppler sonography, the course of the catheter during instillation of fluid is clearly depicted by color coding (Wang 1998).

The inexperienced investigator should practice on models, e.g., on a steak interlarded with olives, or in a water bath. (Mathis 1999)

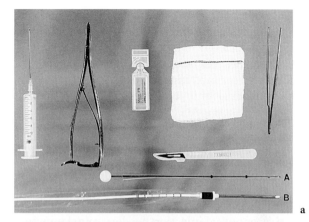

a

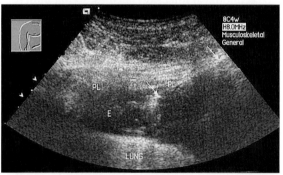

b

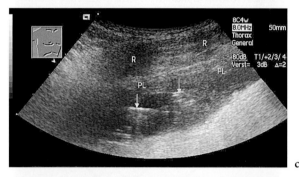

c

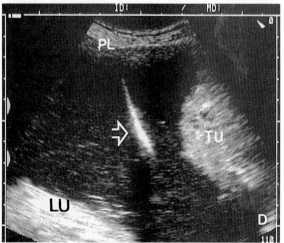

d

Fig. 9.7 a–d. Pleura drainage set (Trokar technique). **a** Thin (12-F) Pneumocath catheter (Intra) (*A*); Trokar catheter (Argyle) (*B*). **b** Sonographically controlled pleura drainage of pleura empyema. The drainage has to be delineated when it is being introduced (Trokar) as a straight, echogenic reflex with sound shadows (*arrows*). *PL*, pleura; *E*, empyema. **c** When the Trokar has been removed, the soft drainage will be hard to discern with sonography because of its twisting course (*arrows*). *R*, ribs. **d** In an echo-free environment (a malign pleura effusion) a drainage is far easier to recognize (*arrow*). *TU*, pleural mesothelioma; *PL*, parietal pleura; *LU*, compressed lung; *D*, diaphragm

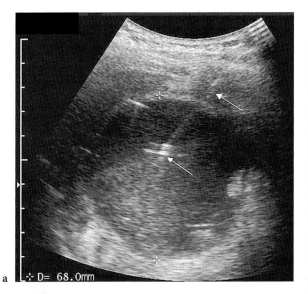

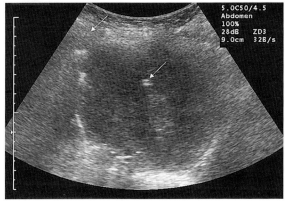

Preparation and Execution of Puncture

As in every intervention, the patient must be informed about the execution and risks of the procedure. The sonographic chest status should be obtained. After the puncture target has been determined, the site, direction, and access of puncture are accurately defined. The non-sterile ultrasound gel is removed. In cases of diagnostic puncture, the investigator should use sterile gloves, local disinfectant spray, and sterile catheter gel if necessary. The patient is positioned such that the focus is optimally accessed. Local anesthesia is only required in cases of multiple puncture or needles with a thick lumen. During puncture, the patient must be asked to briefly hold his breath.

Therapeutic puncture and drainage should be performed in rooms that are wiped daily with disinfectant (Sonnenberg et al. 1998).

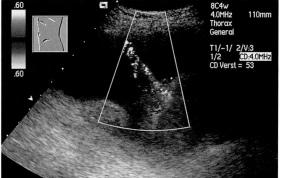

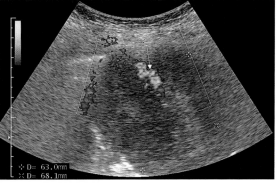

Fig. 9.8. a The needle shaft can be depicted at a great angle (45–90°) as an echogenic, straight-line reflex (*arrows*). The needle tip appears as an echogenic double reflex (*second arrow*, far from the sound head), but only if the needle is being guided correctly at the sound level. Encapsulated pleura empyema (*crosses*). **b** Echogenic double reflex of the needle tip: double reflex, *arrow* far from the sound head. As is so often the case, the puncture was not possible at exactly the sound level. The needle shaft could only be indicated by wobbling movements (*arrow* close to the sound head). Low-echo tumor on the thorax wall. Peripheral bronchial carcinoma (squamous epithelium)

▶

Fig. 9.9. a Color Doppler sonography allows liquid movements in the needle to be detected. The exit of the liquid at the tip of the needle can be seen as a cloud of color. **b** Tissue shifts in the region of the needle tip (slight movement of the needle, or caused by suction) can also be detected by color-Doppler sonography (power Doppler) (*arrow*). Peripheral bronchial carcinoma (*crosses*)

9.3
Indications

Processes of the Chest Wall

Soft tissue tumors should be punctured parallel to the surface of the lung as far as possible. The needle can then be (at a suitable angle) nearly completely imaged in its length and the risk of pneumothorax is minimized (Fig. 9.10).

Needles with a large caliber may be used for this technique (1.4–2 mm). By doing so, even benign lesions are better differentiated (Gleeson et al. 1990; Bradley and Metreweli 1991; Sistrom 1997).

Postoperative accumulation of fluid is treated by multiple puncture or, if necessary, with drainage.

Bone biopsies belong to the domain of computer-assisted puncture when the cortical layer is intact. However, in the presence of cortical defects, even inflammatory or malignant bone lesions can be detected and punctured with sonography (Fig. 9.11). Fine needle aspiration cytology achieves a success rate of 88%–100%. Tumors in the upper thorax aperture can be safely punctured under color-Doppler sonography control (Vogel 1993; Civardi et al. 1994; Blank 1995).

Pleural Cavity

Thoracentesis

In cases of large quantities of effusion, sonography helps to establish the extent of the effusion and to mark the site of puncture in the optimal inter-costal space. The puncture is then performed on the ward (Reuß 1996). In cases of complex effusions (small, loculated, encapsulated, inconvenient location), the puncture is safer when performed under continuous sonographic visual control (Fig. 9.12). In this way, the rate of pneumothorax is markedly reduced (less than 1%) (Yang et al. 1992). The success rate is 97% (O'Moore et al. 1987). Unsuccessful punctures can be avoided when "the fluid color sign" is demonstrated (Fig. 9.13) (Wu et al. 1995). Synthetic indwelling catheters should be given preference over metal ones because of the risk of injury to the lung from metal.

Technique. After applying local anesthesia, the synthetic tube is pushed forward at the upper margin of the rib up to the pleura with a mandrel

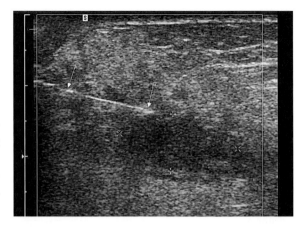

Fig. 9.10. Thorax wall metastasis (*crosses*). The needle shaft (*arrows*) can be delineated very well at this favorable angle

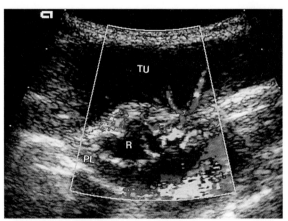

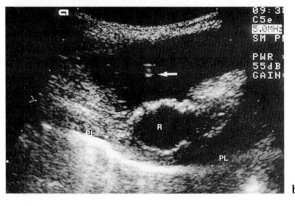

Fig. 9.11. **a** Destroyed rib (*R*). Echo-free "soft-part tumor" (*TU*). Color-Doppler sonography allows vessels to be depicted in the destroyed rib and in the surrounding soft-part tumor. *PL*, pleura. **b** Fine-needle puncture of the soft-part tumor. The tip of the needle can be seen as an echogenic double reflex (*arrow*). Cytology: plasmocytoma. *R*, rib; *PL*, pleura

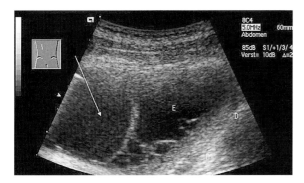

Fig. 9.12. Septate pleural effusion (*E*). Primary diagnostic puncture to obtain an encapsulated empyema (*arrow*). The secondary step involved pleura drainage. *D*, diaphragm

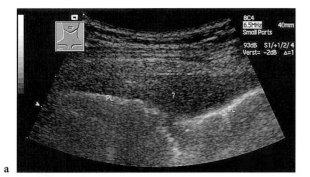

a

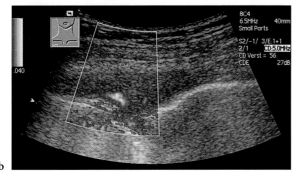

b

Fig. 9.13. a B-scan sonography for a differential diagnosis of an encapsulated effusion or fresh thickening. *PL*, visceral pleura. **b** Power Doppler demonstrates advanced vascularization with high-caliber vessels. Fresh pleural thickening

Uncomplicated pleural effusions in the presence of cardiac insufficiency and even small pneumothoraces after puncture can be treated with thoracentesis.

Malignant pleural effusions, accumulation of pus or blood should be treated with a drain because of the risk of septation (Blank 1994).

The success rate of cytology in malignant effusions is no more than 50%–75% (Gartmann 1988). In tuberculous effusions, pathogens are demonstrated in only 20%–40% (Vladutiu 1986). Since even the classical pleural blind biopsy according to Abrams or Ramell has an accuracy of no more than 50% in malignant effusions, video-assisted thoracoscopy is used increasingly often. Sonography-guided pleural biopsy is one alternative. However, the procedure has been used in a very small number of cases so far (Müller et al. 1988). The recently introduced forceps biopsy needles might be helpful (Fig. 9.14) (Seitz 1999). Fine needle aspiration biopsy of tissue taken from a pleural thick-

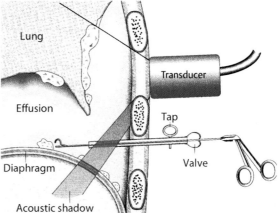

a

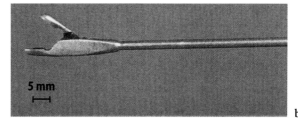

b

Fig. 9.14. a The pleural forceps biopsy according to Seitz. **b** Pleural biopsy forceps according to Seitz (Storz Medical Equipment, Tuttlingen)

(Abbocath; Abbott, Abbott Park, Ill.). Entry into the pleura is marked by a mild increase in resistance. The mandrel is then removed. In a closed system, special pleural drainage sets can be used to perform manual aspiration.

ening is of no value and is even hazardous. It may only be employed in the presence of focal lesions (Mathis 1999a).

Percutaneous Pleural Drainage

Given the appropriate indication, malignant, hemorrhagic, and inflammatory pleural effusions may be treated with a sonography-guided pleural drain. In cases of malignant effusions, catheters with a narrow lumen [7–12 F, e.g., Pleurocath (Plastimed)] will suffice. The puncture is usually performed using the trocar technique. The catheter is placed in the deepest site of the pleural cavity.

Early diagnostic verification of a *pleural empyema* is important, as percutaneous therapy is only successful (success rate, 72%–88%) in the acute phase (weeks 1–4) (Fig. 9.15) (Klose and Günther 1988; Blank 1994). The success of drainage in the presence of septation can be markedly improved by the instillation of urokinase (50–100,000 IU per treatment; Sistrom 1997).

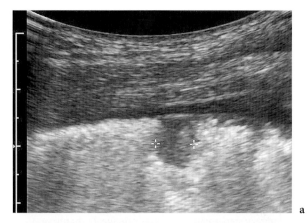
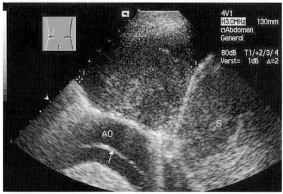

Fig. 9.16. a Several small peripheral lung tumors (maximum diameter, 18 mm) located on the thorax wall. Mild pleura effusion. Fine-needle aspiration cytology revealed small-cell bronchial carcinoma. **b** Large mass, left dorsobasal location (*crosses*), alongside the diaphragm and also the aorta descendens (*AO*). A dissecting aortic aneurysm had been identified in this patient 4 years earlier. Dissection membrane (*arrow*). Fine-needle incision biopsy (Sonocan needle, 0.9 mm in diameter). Histology: squamous cell carcinoma. *S*, spleen

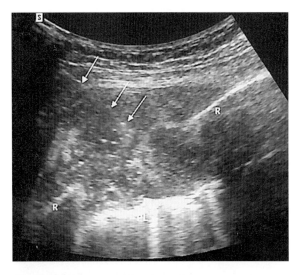

Fig. 9.15. An 80-year-old patient, whose temperature rose rapidly a few days after a fall which caused an injury to the left side of the thorax. X-ray reveals a shadow located on the thorax wall, and raises the suspicion of a fractured rib. Sonographic mass with infiltration into the thorax wall. Minor fluid movements were perceptible during the dynamic examination. Diagnostic puncture was unsuccessful until a coarse needle (diameter, 2 mm) was used. Needle shaft (*arrows*). It proved possible to extract highly viscous pus. This was followed by pleural drainage. *R*, rib

Lung Consolidations

At the time of diagnosis, two thirds of lung carcinomas are no longer curable by surgery. The histological type must be determined before palliative therapeutic measures are employed. In the diagnosis of the peripheral lung tumor, sonography-guided puncture is markedly superior to bronchoscopy, much easier and faster to perform than radiography or even computer-assisted percutaneous biopsy, and without of radiation (Fig. 9.16a, b) (Chandrasekhar et al. 1976; Börner 1986; O'Moore et al. 1987; Hsu et al. 1996). Using fine-needle punc-

Table 9.4. Sonography-guided chest puncture: accuracy and rate of pneumothorax

Author	Year	Patients (n)	Accuracy (%)	Pneumothorax (%)
Izumi	1982	20	80	0
Schwerk	1982	15	93	0.5
Cinti	1984	12	83	0
Ikezoe	1984	38	79	0
Yang	1985	25	84	8
Pedersen et al.	1986	45	84	2
Pang	1987	54	85	4
Heckemann	1988	42	98	6
Yin	1989	85	98	2.4
Ikezoe et al.	1990	124	90/67	4
Bradley	1991	30	90	0
Mikloweit et al.	1991	45	85	4.4
Targhetta	1992	64	86	3
Schulz	1992	75	91	2.5
Yang et al.	1992	218	95	1.3
Yuan	1992	30	92/83[a]	3
Metz	1993	41	84.6	5
Tikkakoski	1993	200	93	2.5
Chu	1994	116	92/53	?
Czwerwenka	1994	82	83	0
Vogel	1995	110	70	3.6
Hsu et al.	1996	188	94	1.6
Knudsen	1996	128	93	4
Beckh and Bölcskei	1997	50	92	2
Dallari	1999	45	92/33	?
Mathis	1999	155	92/87[a]	1.9
Total		1876		2.6

[a] Malignant/benign lesions.

ture (histology), an accuracy of 70%–90% is achieved in cases of carcinoma and metastases (Table 9.4) (Mathis and Gehmacher 1999). Peripheral tumors <3 cm in size can be better diagnosed by fine needle aspiration cytology (Sistrom 1997). Fine-needle puncture is not always sufficient (accuracy, 70%) to distinguish benign tumors. Wedge resections obtained by thoracoscopy are preferred in many cases (Beckh 1997).

Lung Abscesses

Even small pulmonary abscesses that escape detection on X-ray can be imaged by sonography (6–7 mm). If antibiotic therapy does not yield the desired result, fluid may be aspirated from the region of the abscess under sonographic guidance. By this means, the pathogen can be isolated in 65% of cases (Gehmacher 1996). If therapy continues

to fail, lung abscess drainage may be performed under sonographic guidance (Fig. 9.17) (Sonnenberg 1991; Klein 1995). The risk of fistula formation is minimized when the investigator uses the shortest access and traverses solid, homogeneous, infiltrated, or atelectatic tissue (Mathis 1999).

Mediastinum

Few space-occupying masses in the mediastinum (retrosternal goiter, cyst, aneurysm, thrombosis) can be reliably classified on the basis of characteristic sonographic features. An investigation of fine tissue is needed in order to determine the etiology of the lesion. Gentle removal of tissue without causing a large defect is very important in the diagnosis of space-occupying masses that can be removed by surgery (Rosenberg 1993). Therefore, puncture under imaging guidance should be the

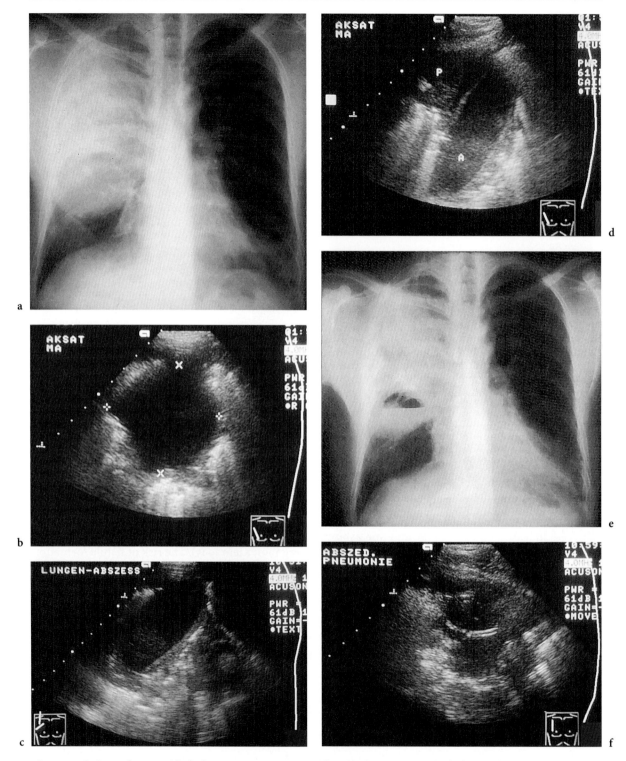

Fig. 9.17 a–f. Lung abscess with drainage. **a** A young man with typical pneumonia. **b–d** Abscess formation not seen in early first chest X-ray. *A*, abscess; *P*, pneumonia. **e** Abscess cavern in chest X-ray. **f** US-guided drainage

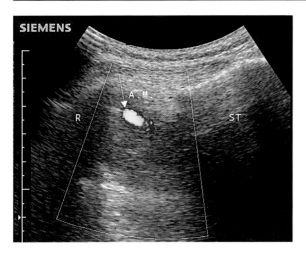

Fig. 9.18. Mediastinal tumor. Parasternal plumb line in the right lateral position. Low-echo, indistinctly delineated mass (located in the color window). Color-Doppler sonography in "power" mode shows the parasternally located mammary vessels, which have to be preserved from harm during a punch biopsy. *R*, rib; *AM*, arteria mammaria; *ST*, sternum

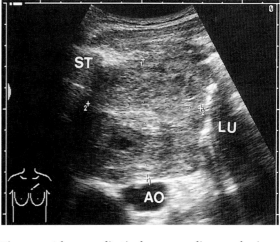

Fig. 9.19. A large mediastinal mass was discovered primarily by sonography, located parasternally left, in a 19-year-old patient during emergency treatment connected with an upper inflow congestion. A punch biopsy was carried out immediately (Sonocan needle, 1.2 mm in diameter). Histologically, a highly malignant non-Hodgkin lymphoma was diagnosed. *ST*, sternum; *LU*, lung; *AO*, aorta descendens

first procedure. When this is done, space-occupying masses in the mediastinum can be easily punctured from a suprasternal or parasternal approach under sonographic guidance (Nordenstrom 1967; Rubens et al. 1997). The rate of accuracy is 54%–100%, the rate of complications, 0–4%. Vessels should be avoided (color-Doppler sonography) (Fig. 9.18) (Blank et al. 1996). In cases of superficial lesions (thymomas, lymphomas), gross needles are given preference. Using a needle with a thick lumen, correct histological classification is achieved in up to 93% of cases and the rate of complications is only slightly higher (less than 1%) (Fig. 9.19). In contrast to radiographic or computed tomography-guided puncture (10%–44%), a pneumothorax is rarely encountered (Yang et al. 1992; Heilo 1993, 1996; Schuler et al. 1995; Gupta 1998).

In recent years, endosonographic transesophageal guided puncture has also been used successfully. It is a good complement to percutaneous puncture, as lesions in the anterior mediastinum are not easily accessed, in contrast to those in the posterior and lower mediastinum (Schlotterbeck et al. 1997; Pedersen et al. 1996; Hüner et al. 1998; Janssen et al. 1998).

9.4
Risks

Sonography-guided puncture has a low rate of complications. The rate of pneumothorax is 2.8%; 1% requires drainage (Table 9.4). Hemorrhage or hemoptysis is observed in 0%–2%. Data concerning air embolism or even death are not available so far. Tumor dissemination through the procedure of puncture (vaccine metastases) is of little clinical significance and very rare (less than 0.003%). In cases of malignant pleural mesothelioma, it is slightly more common. When surgery is performed, the puncture site is also resected (Weiss and Düntsch 1996; Mathis 1999).

Pneumothorax After Puncture

If the focus is no longer visible after the puncture, the likelihood of a pneumothorax is high. This can be reliably detected by sonography, through the absence of respiration-dependent gliding movement of the pleura (Fig. 9.20) (Wernecke et al. 1989; Blank 1994).

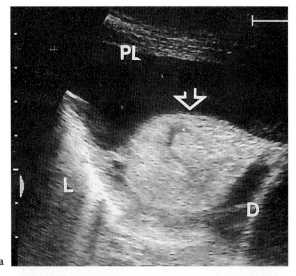

a

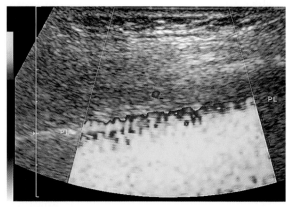

c

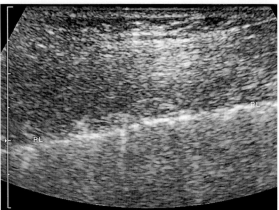

b

Fig. 9.20. a A blood coagulum (*arrow*) presenting as a complication following diagnostic pleural effusion puncture. *PL*, parietal pleura; *L*, compressed lung; *D*, diaphragm. **b** A pneumothorax was excluded by showing the sliding sign of the pleura. *PL*, parietal pleura. **c** Color-Doppler sonography in "power" mode allowed the respiration-dependent sliding sign to be documented impressively even in the static image. The repeat echoes that could be demonstrated with B-scan sonography (artifact) dorsal to the lung surface accordingly show up as a color artifact. This cannot be demonstrated in cases of pneumothorax. *PL*, parietal pleura

The quantity of free air can only be measured by obtaining a chest radiograph. A pneumothorax usually reaches its maximum dimensions after 3 h, so that the decision regarding a therapeutic procedure is made thereafter, when the pneumothorax is small. If the patient is symptomatic, or if a larger volume is present, the patient is initially given protracted thoracentesis. The success rate within the first 10 h is 90% (Klose 1996). In the event of renewed collapse, the clinician should use a percutaneous drain and a catheter with a small lumen. A routine chest radiograph is not required after sonography-guided puncture.

Summary

Provided the indication is established with care, interventional measures in the thorax are very successful. The rate of complications is low when the procedure is performed by trained therapists. The basic principle to be applied is: "Try ultrasound first" (Sistrom 1997).

Acknowledgments. I would like to express my thanks to Professor Lenz (chief consultant surgeon in the Radiology Department of the Steinenberg Clinic, Reutlingen) for preparing and providing the radiological findings, and to Mr. Klinkmüller and my son Valentin for the technical photographic work.

References

Beckh S, Bölcskei PL (1997) Biopsie thorakaler Raumforderungen – Von der computertomographischen zur ultraschallgezielten Punktion. Ultraschall Med 18:220–225

Blank W (1994) Sonographisch gesteuerte Punktionen und Drainagen. In: Braun B, Günther R, Schwerk WB (Hrsg) Ultraschalldiagnostik. Lehrbuch und Atlas. ecomed, Landsberg/Lech, III-11.1:1–79

Blank W (1995) Weichteil- und Knochentumoren. In: Braun B, Günther R, Schwerk WB (Hrsg) Ultraschalldiagnostik. Lehrbuch und Atlas. ecomed, Landsberg/Lech, III-9.9:1–27

Blank W, Schuler A, Wild K, Braun B (1996) Transthoracic sonography of the mediastinum. Europ J Ultrasound 3:179–190

Börner N (1986) Sonographische Diagnostik pleuropulmonaler Erkrankungen. Med Klin 81:496–500

Bradley MJ, Metreweli C (1991) Ultrasound in the diagnosis of the juxta-pleural lesion. Brit J Radiol 64:330–333

Braun B (1983) Abdominelle und thorakale Ultraschalldiagnostik. In: Bock HE, Gerok W, Hartmann F et al. (Hrsg) Klinik der Gegenwart. Urban & Schwarzenberg, München, S 1141–1145

Chandresakar AJ, Reynes CJ, Churchill RJ (1976) Ultrasonically guided transthoracic percutaneous biopsy of peripheral pulmonary masses. Chest 70:627–630

Chu CY Hsu WH, Hsu JY, Huang CM, Shih CM, Chiang DC (1994) Ultrasound-guided biopsy of thoracic masses. Chung Hua I Hsueh Tsa Chih 54:336–342

Cinti D, Hawkins HB (1984) Aspiration biopsy of peripheral pulmonary masses using real-time sonographic guidance. Am J Roentgenol 142:1115–1116

Civardi G, Livraghi T, Colombo MD (1994) Lytic bone lesions suspected for metastasis: ultrasonically guided fine-needle aspiration biopsy. J Clin Ultrasound 22:307–311

Ckzerwenka W, Otto RC (1994) Die ultraschallgezielte Lungenpunktion. Bildgebung Imaging 61 (S2): 12

Dallari R, Gollini C, Barozzi G, Gilioli F (1999) Ultrasound-guided percutaneous needle aspiration biopsy of peripheral pumonary lesions. Monaldi Arch Chest Dis 54: 7–10

Gartmann JC (1988) Der unklare Pleuraerguß: Praktisch-diagnostisches Vorgehen. Therapeutische Umschau 45:308–313

Gehmacher O, Mathis G, Kopf A, Scheier M (1996) Ultrasound imaging of pneumonia. Ultrasound Med Biol 21: 1119–1122

Gleeson F, Lomas DJ, Flower CDR, Stewart S (1990) Powered cutting needle biopsy of the pleura and chest wall. Clin Radiol 41:199–200

Gupta S, Gulati M, Rajwanski A, Gupta P, Suri S (1998) Sonographically guided fine-needle aspiration biopsy of superior mediastinal lesions by the suprasternal route. AJR 171:1303–1306

Heckemann R, Hohner S, Heutz J, Nakhosten J (1988) Ultraschallgeführte Feinnadelpunktion solider pulmonaler und pleuraler Tumoren. Ultraschall Klin Prax S1:83

Heilo A (1993) Tumors in the mediastinum: US-guided histologic core-needle biopsy. Radiology 189:143–146

Heilo A (1996) US-guided transthoracic biopsy. Europ J Ultrasound 3:141–153

Hsu WH, Chiang DC, Hsu JY, Kwan PC, Chen CL, Chen DY (1996) Ultrasound guided fine-needle aspiration biopsy of lung cancers. J Clin Ultrasound 24:225–233

Hüner M, Ghadim BM, Haensch W, Schlag DM (1998) Transesophageal biopsy of mediastinal and pulmonary tumors by means of endoscopic ultrasound guidance. J Thorac Cardic Vascular Surgery 116:554–559

Ikezoe J, Sone S, Higashihara T, Morimoto S, Arisawa J, Kuriiyama K (1984) Sonographically guided needle biopsy for diagnosis of thoracic lesions. Amer J Roentgenol 143:229–243

Ikezoe J, Morimoto S, Arisawa J, Takasgima S, Kozuka T, Nakahara K (1990) Percutaneous biopsy of thoracic lesions: value of sonography for needle guidance. Am J Roentgenol 154:1181–1185

Izumi S, Tamaki S, Natori H, Kira S (1982) Ultrasonically guided aspiration needle biopsy in diseases of the chest. Am Rev Respir Dis 125:460–464

Janssen J, Johann W, Luis W, Greiner L (1998) Zum klinischen Stellenwert der endosonographisch gesteuerten transoesophagealen Feinnadelpunktion von Mediastinalprozessen. Dtsch Med Wochenschr 123:1402–1409

Kelbel C, Stephany P, Lorenz J (1996) Endoluminal chest sonography. Europ J Ultrasound 3:191–195

Klein JS, Schultz S, Heffner JE (1995) Interventional radiology of the chest: image-guided percutaneous drainage of pleural effusions, lung abscess, and pneumothorax. AJR 164:581–588

Klose KC, Günther RW (1996) CT-gesteuerte Punktionen. In: Günther RW, Thelen M (Hrsg) Interventionelle Radiologie. Thieme, Stuttgart, S 750–775

Knudsen DU, Nielsen SM, Hariri J, Christersen J, Kristersen S (1996) Ultrasonographically guided fine-needle aspiration biopsy of intrathoracic tumors. Acta Radiol 37: 327–331

Mathis G (1997a) Thoraxsonography – Part I: Chest Wall and Pleura. Ultrasound Med Biol, 23/8:1131–1139

Mathis G (1997b) Thoraxsonography – Part II: Peripheral Pulmonary Consolidation. Ultrasound Med Biol, 23/8: 1141–1153

Mathis G, Bitschnau R, Gehmacher O, Dirschmid K (1999) Ultraschallgeführte transthorakale Punktion. Ultraschall Med 20:226–235

Mathis G, Gehmacher O (1999) Ultrasound-guided diagnostic and therapeutic interventions in peripheral pulmonary masses. Wien Klin Wochenschr 111:230–235

Metz V, Dock W, Zyhlarz R, Eibenberger K, Farres MT, Grabenwöger F (1993) Ultraschallgezielte Nadelbiopsien thorakaler Raumforderungen. ROFO 159:60–63

Mikloweit P, Zachgo W, Lörcher U, Meier-Sydow J (1991) Pleuranahe Lungenprozesse: Diagnostische Wertigkeit Sonographie versus Computertomographie (CT). Bildgebung 58:127–131

Mueller PR, Sanjay S, Simeone JF et al. (1988) Image-guided pleural biopsies: Indications, technique and results in 23 patients. Radiology 169:1–4

Nordenstrom B (1967) Paraxiphoid approach to mediastinum for mediastinography and mediastinal needle biopsy: a preliminary report. Invest Radiol 2:141–146

O'Moore PV, Mueller PR, Simeone JF, Saini S, Butch RJ, Hahn PF (1987) Sonographic guidance in diagnostic and therapeutic interventions in the pleural space. AJR 149:1–5

Pang JA, Tsang MB, Hom L, Metreweli C (1987) Ultrasound guided tissue-core biopsy of thoracic lesions with trucut and surecut needles. Chest 91:823–828

Pedersen BH, Vilmann P, Folke K, Jacobsen GK, Krasnik M, Milman N, Hancke S (1996) Endoscopic ultrasonography and real-time guided fine-needle aspiration biopsy of solid lesions of the mediastinum suspected of malignancy. Chest 110:539–544

Pedersen OM, Aasen TB, Gulsvik A (1986) Fine needle aspiration biopsy of mediastinal and peripheral pulmonary masses guided by real time sonography. Chest 89:504–508

Reuß J (1996) Sonographic imaging of the pleura: nearly 30 years experience. Europ J Ultrasound 3:125–139

Rosenberg JC (1993) Neoplasms of the mediastinum. In: De Vita VT, Hellmann S, Rosenberg SA (eds) Cancer: principles & practice of oncology. Lippincott, Philadelphia, pp 759–775

Rubens DJ, Strang JG, Fultz PJ, Gottleib RH (1997) Sonographic guidance of mediastinal biopsy: an effective alternative to CT guidance. AJR 169:1605–1610

Schlotterbeck K, Schmid J, Klein F, Alber G (1997) Transesophageal sonography in the staging of lung cancer. Ultraschall Med 18:153–158

Schuler A, Blank W, Braun B (1995) Sonographisch-interventionelle Diagnostik bei Thymomen. Ultraschall Med 16:62

Schulz G (1992) Interventionelle Thoraxsonographie bei brustwandnahen soliden Raumforderungen. Ultraschall Klin Prax 7:202

Schwerk WB, Dombrowski H, Kalbfleisch H (1982) Ultraschalltomographie und gezielte Feinnadelbiopsie intrathorakaler Raumforderungen. Ultraschall Med 3:212–218

Schwerk WB, Görg C (1993) Pleura und Lunge. In: Braun B, Günther R, Schwerk WB (Hrsg) Ultraschalldiagnostik. Lehrbuch und Atlas. ecomed, Landsberg/Lech, III-2.2: 1–44

Seitz K, Pfeffer A, Littmann M, Seitz G (1999) Sonographisch gesteuerte Zangenbiopsie der Pleura. Ultraschall Med 20:60–65

Sistrom CI (1997) Thoracic Sonography for Diagnosis and Intervention. Curr Probl Diagn Radiol January/February 1:6–46

Sonnenberg E, Agostino H, Casola G, Wittich GR, Varney RR, Harker C (1991) Lung abscess: CT-guided drainage. Radiology 178:347–351

Sonnenberg E, Wittich GR, Goodacre BW, Zwischenberger JB (1998) Percutaneous drainage of thoracic collections. J Thorac Imaging 13:74–82

Targhetta R, Bourgeois JM, Chavagneux R, Balmes P (1992) Diagnosis of pneumothorax by ultrasound immediately after ultrasonically guided aspiration biopsy. Chest 101:855–856

Tikkakoski T, Lohela P, Taavitsainen M et al. (1993) Transthoracic lesions: diagnosis by ultrasound-guided biopsy. ROFO 159:444–449

Vladutiu AO (1986) Pleural effusion. Mount Kisco, Futura Publishing, New York

Vogel B (1985) Ultraschallgezielte perthorakale Punktion. Prax Klin Pneumol 39:632–635

Vogel B (1993) Ultrasonographic detection and guided biopsy of thoracic osteolysis. Chest 104:1003–1005

Wang HC, Yu DJ, Yang PC (1995) Transthoracic needle biopsy of thoracic tumor by Color Doppler ultrasound puncture guided device. Thorax 50:1258–1263

Weiss H, Weiss A (1994) Therapeutische interventionelle Sonographie. Ultraschall Med 15:152–158

Weiss H, Düntsch U (1996) Komplikationen der Feinnadelbiopsie – DEGUM-Umfrage II. Ultraschall Med 17:118–130

Wernecke K, Galanski M, Peters PE, Hansen J (1989) Pneumothorax: Sonographische Diagnostik des Pneumothorax. Fortschr Röntgenstr 150:84–85

Westcott JL (1980) Direct percutaneous needle aspiration of localized pulmonary lesions: Result in 422 patients. Radiology 137:31–35

Wu RG, Yang PC, Kuo SH, Luh KT (1995) "Fluid color" sign: a useful indicator for discrimination between pleural thickening and pleural effusion. J Ultrasound Med 14:767–769

Yang PC (1996) Color Doppler ultrasound of pulmonary consolidation. Europ J Ultrasound 3:169–178

Yang PC, Luh KT, Sheu JC, Kuo SH, Sang SP (1985) Peripheral pulmonary lesions: ultrasonography and ultrasonically guided aspiration biopsy. Radiology 155:451–456

Yang PC, Chang DB, Yu CJ, Lee YC, Kuo SH, Luh KT (1992) Ultrasound-guided core biopsy of thoracic tumors. Amer Rev Respir Dis 146:763–767

Yin XJ (1989) Ultrasound-guided percutaneous needle biopsy in diseases of the chest. Chung Hua Wai Ko Tsa Chih 27:107–108

Yuan A, Yang PC, Chang DB, Yu CJ, Lee YC, Kuo SH, Luh KT (1992) Ultrasound-guided aspiration biopsy of small peripheral pulmonary nodules. Chest 101:926–930

10 Stepwise Diagnostic Imaging Procedures in Pneumology

S. BECKH

The value of specific imaging methods for various lung diseases in which imaging procedures significantly contribute to the diagnosis is discussed. The procedure for pulmonary embolism is detailed in Chap. 4, Sect. 4.3. In some cases, the sequence of investigations is dependent on the availability of equipment, the condition of the patient, and the experience of the physician.

10.1 Chest Pain

The flexibility with which ultrasonography can be applied permits fast, symptom-based diagnosis in cases of *chest pain* (Fig. 10.1).

The probe is placed directly on the site of maximum pain or the site of physical examination. Rib fractures and concomitant hematomas can be easily detected (Dubs-Kunz 1996; Mathis 1997a; Fig. 10.2).

The localization of a pathological finding in the case of radiating pain is somewhat more difficult. Quite often, a persistent "cervical spine" or a "shoulder-arm syndrome" conceals a Pancoast tumor (Rapoport et al. 1988; Padovani et al. 1993; Arcasoy and Jett 1997; Fig. 10.3).

Sonography will clearly show the invasive infiltration of muscle. However, to assess the extent of such infiltration in vertebrae and the spinal canal, survey radiographs and special sectional images are required (Fig. 10.4).

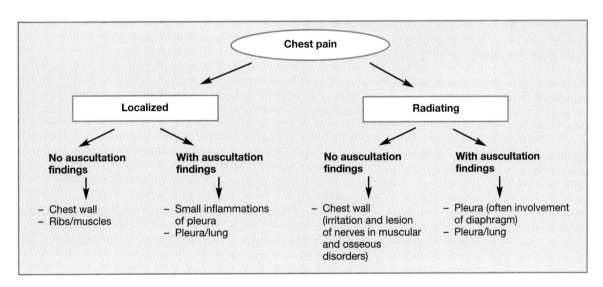

Fig. 10.1. Chest pain and auscultation as an orientation for targeted sonographic investigation

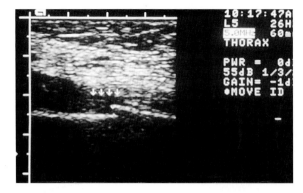

Fig. 10.2. On the right side, in the posterior axillary line, a mildly dislocated fracture of the 9th rib with hematoma (*arrows*) above the site of fracture. After severe coughing attacks, the patient, who was under anticoagulant therapy, complained of chest pain in the right side. Simultaneously, a hematoma occurred in the soft tissue on the right side of the chest. The fact that the site of fracture was the cause of the hematoma had escaped detection on radiographs and CT

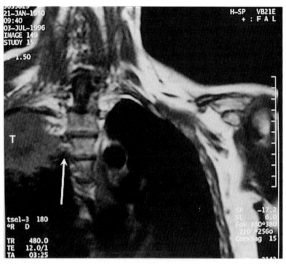

Fig. 10.4. Magnetic resonance tomography in a Pancoast tumor (squamous cell carcinoma) of the right upper lobe, previously diagnosed by sonographic biopsy. Tumor branches (*arrow*) infiltrate the vertebral column and the spinal canal. *T*, tumor

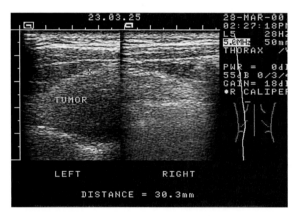

Fig. 10.3. On the left side, dorsal, apical and paravertebral, a hypoechoic space-occupying mass. Compared to the healthy side, the tumor clearly infiltrates the neck muscles through the left dome of the pleura into the neck muscles. Sonographic biopsy: moderately differentiated, mildly keratinizing squamous cell carcinoma

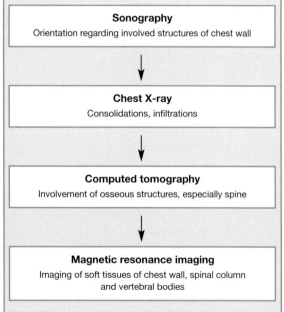

Fig. 10.5. Diagnostic imaging in the presence of chest pain

In cases of painful inflammatory lung and pleural disease, sonography may well be the foremost imaging procedure. However, a chest radiograph remains indispensable for obtaining an overview (Fig. 10.5).

10.2
Pleural Disease

The spectrum of pleural disease includes the following entities:

- Pleuritis
- Pleural effusion, "white lung"
- Empyema
- Pleural carcinomatosis
- Tumor:
  - Benign (lipoma, solitary fibrous tumor)
  - Mesothelioma

Sonography may well be used as the primary diagnostic procedure (Morris and Wiggins 1992; Fraser et al. 1999 a). It is a fast source of information for:

- Documenting pleural and subpleural foci (Fig. 10.6)
- Distinguishing between liquid and solid foci (Fig. 10.6)
- Imaging a subpulmonary effusion
- Documenting septation of an effusion (Fig. 10.7)
- Evaluating the mobility of the diaphragm and lung in dynamic investigation (Fig. 10.8)
- Imaging vessels (Fig. 10.14)
- Localizing of the optimal site of puncture

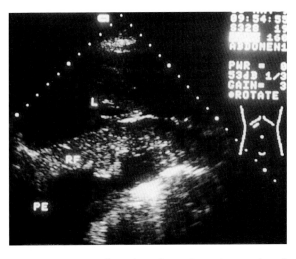

Fig. 10.6. On transhepatic subcostal section, a broad space-occupying mass (tumor) along the entire right dome of the diaphragm, cranial pleural effusion (*PE*). Sonographic biopsy: pleural carcinosis due to an adenoid-cystic carcinoma. *L*, liver

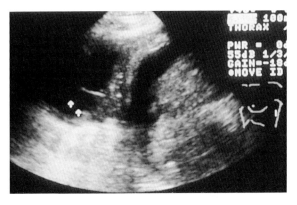

Fig. 10.7. After pleurodesis because of a malignant pleural effusion (metastatic colon carcinoma), the partially ventilated left lower lobe is adherent to the parietal pleura. Above and below this site, a pleural effusion with septa (*arrows*)

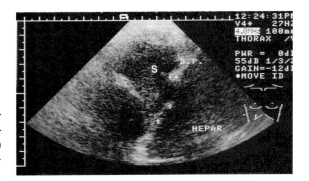

Fig. 10.8. On longitudinal section in the mid-clavicular line, tumor infiltration (*arrows*; *S*, space-occupying mass) of the diaphragm (*D.P.*) by a pleural mesothelioma (histological investigation after sonographic biopsy)

A *survey radiograph* is the next diagnostic step. Additional sectional images with *computed tomography* are useful to evaluate the full extent of pathological changes (Leung et al. 1990; Fraser et al. 1999b; Arenas-Jiménez et al. 2000; Düster et al. 2000) in the following cases:

- Pleural empyema (Fig. 10.9)
- Unclear pleural space-occupying masses
- Pleural mesothelioma (Fig. 10.10)
- Looking for intrapulmonary foci (Fig. 10.11)
- Determining the density of foci (Fig. 10.12)
- Imaging the mediastinum and vessels

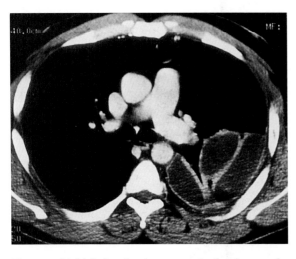

Fig. 10.9. Multiply loculated empyema in the chest on the right side. CT shows the full extent of the finding

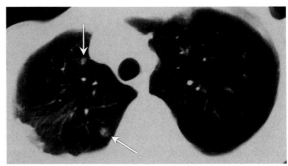

Fig. 10.11. Irregular thickening of the pleura on spiral CT; adenocarcinoma cells were found in the pleural effusion. Additionally, two small intrapulmonary circular foci (*arrows*)

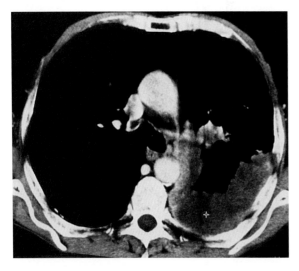

Fig. 10.10. CT of a pleural mesothelioma spreading along the entire dorsal mediastinal pleura

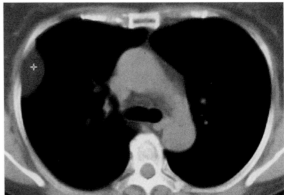

Fig. 10.12. An incidental finding on the radiograph: a peripheral space-occupying mass in the right upper lobe. Sonographically homogeneous, smoothly margined pleural focus. Density measurement on CT clearly showed a pleural lipoma. The patient refused to undergo biopsy

Magnetic resonance tomography should be used in the following cases (Morris and Wiggins 1992; Layer 1998):

- When CT is not possible
- For preoperative staging in the evaluation of:
  - Chest wall infiltration
  - Osseous infiltration (see Fig. 10.4)
  - Infiltration of mediastinal structures

The investigator should be generous in establishing the indication for *bronchoscopy*, so that a central bronchial carcinoma is not overlooked. *Positron emission tomography* (PET) may be useful to distinguish between inflammatory or malignant and inactive cicatricial foci (Knopp and Bischoff 1998). However, a reliable distinction between benign-inflammatory (e.g., tuberculosis) and malignant changes (e.g., mesothelioma) cannot be made. *Thoracoscopy* is known to produce positive results in 95% of cases (Loddenkemper and Boutin 1993). Thus, it provides the maximum diagnostic information but is also the most invasive method.

10.3
Pneumonia

Pneumonia is manifested as an inflammation of the lung parenchyma with characteristic clinical symptoms such as fever, cough, and in cases of pleural infestation, respiration-dependent pain. The extent and nature of infiltration should be investigated with a *survey radiograph* (Fig. 10.13). *Sonography* can be used as a complementary procedure (Mathis 1997b) to document:

- Peripheral infiltration
- A pleural effusion
- An abscess
- An air bronchogram
- To differentiate a solid focus/an infiltration
- The organization of pleuritic pneumonia (Fig. 10.14)

A *computed tomography* is required in cases of:

- Complicated course of disease (Figs. 10.15–10.19)
- Interlobular effusions
- Suspicion of tumor

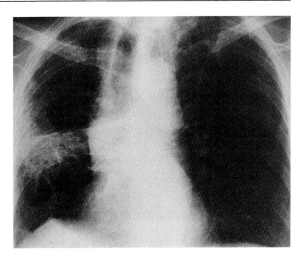

Fig. 10.13. Infiltration of the middle lobe and partially the right upper lobe. Prolonged clinical healing of pneumonia

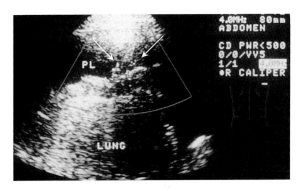

Fig. 10.14. Sonography after 14 days of treatment for pleuritic pneumonia in the right lower lobe (pneumococci) with pleural effusion (*PL*). The radiograph still shows residual shadows in a basal location on the right side. No effusion on sonography, but organization of pleuritic pneumonia with sprouting vessels (*arrows*). The initial intention to puncture the presumed residual effusion was discarded!

Magnetic resonance tomography is less suitable to investigate ventilated portions of the lung because of the low proton density of parenchyma. In cases of complicated solid foci (Agrons et al. 1998), MRI might provide additional diagnostic information. *Endoscopy* should be used to determine pathogens and to inspect the central respiratory tract.

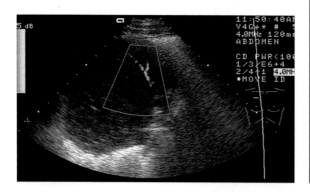

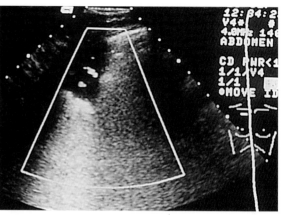

Fig. 10.15. A 37-year-old man with acute, severe disease and high fever. On radiographs (see Fig. 10.17), a large peripheral space-occupying mass in the right upper lobe, raising the suspicion of a tumor. The sonographic finding of a hypoechoic focus with numerous, nearly echo-free necroses and regular branching vessels in the medial aspect is indicative of abscess-forming/necrotizing pneumonia

Fig. 10.16. After 14 days of treatment, the entity is smaller on sonography. However, a broad, non-mobile air reflex is seen from the lateral aspect, raising the suspicion of a large colliquation. Vessels in the medial aspect are unaltered

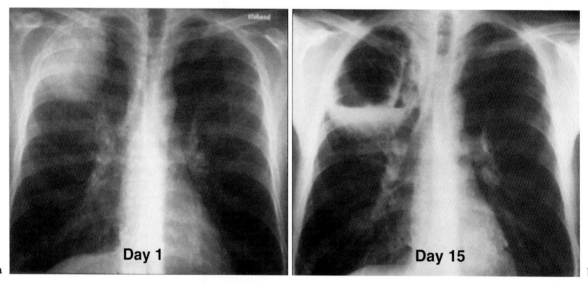

a   b

Fig. 10.17 a, b. Corresponding course of survey radiographs relating to Figs. 10.15 (a) and 10.16 (b)

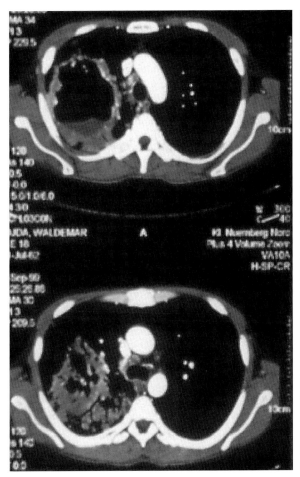

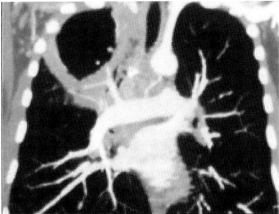

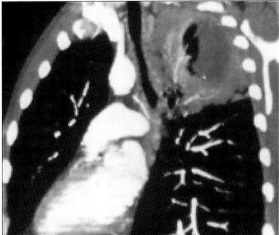

Fig. 10.18. On CT, corresponding to the sonogram in Fig. 10.16, a large colliquation with marginal vessels, which can be followed as accessory upper lobe arteries up to the pulmonary artery. Because of the risk of fatal bleeding due to sudden rupture of the marginal vessels, resection of the upper lobe was performed. Necrotizing pneumonia was confirmed

Fig. 10.19. Clinically, serologically, and histologically established Wegener's disease with pulmonary foci at the time of diagnosis. On both sides, CT shows dense foci with blurred margins and fine ramifications into the lung parenchyma. The foci resolved well under treatment with prednisolone and cyclophosphamide ▶

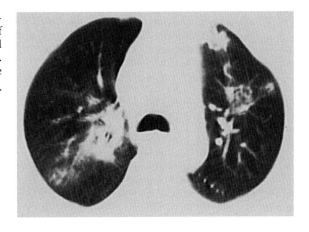

10.4
Diffuse Pulmonary Disease

In cases of diffuse pulmonary disease *sonography* plays a minor role. It is able to demonstrate the following entities:

- Callus formation
- Calcareous plaques
- Asbestos plaques (Fig. 10.20)
- Effusion
- Solid peripheral space-occupying masses

On the lung surface, one finds uncharacteristic scars or uneven marginal contours (Fig. 10.21), such as those frequently observed in cases of chronic obstructive respiratory disease or after pleuritic pneumonia.

A ground-breaking diagnostic procedure is *high-resolution computed tomography* (HRCT; Swensen et al. 1997; Vahlensieck 1998; Reynolds 1998; Fig. 10.22), which, along with survey radiographs, is also the method of choice for evaluating the disease course.

When diffuse pulmonary disease is suspected, the following procedure should be adopted (modified according to the German Society of Pneumology, 1994):

- Survey radiograph in two planes
- Sonography aimed at clarifying the specific issue under investigation (see above), echocardiography
- Investigation of lung function at rest and during exercise, if necessary with inhalational provocation testing
- Special serological tests (e.g., ACE, antinuclear factors, ANCA, rheumatism serology, precipitins of type III allergies)
- HRCT to evaluate:
  - Disease activity
  - The nature of disease
  - Selection of the most suitable biopsy site
  - Course
- Bronchoscopy for:
  - Peribronchial biopsy
  - Bronchoalveolar lavage
- Thoracoscopic biopsy

10.5
Pulmonary Nodule

A circular pulmonary focus is usually an incidental radiographic finding in an entirely asymptomatic patient. Comparison studies with computed tomography, especially spiral CT, have shown that up to 50 % of foci less than 10 mm in size, especially those in the periphery of the lung, the hilum of the lung, in retrocardiac location, and in the phrenicocostal angle, escape detection on survey radiographs (Heindel 1998). The imaging procedures listed in Fig. 10.23 contribute to the diagnostic work-up (Remy-Jardin et al. 1993; Munden et al. 1997; Rozenshtein et al. 1998 Tuengerthal 1998).

Fluoroscopy may help to exclude false foci (shadow of the mamilla) and overlapping artifacts, or may be used for targeted localization of deep pulmonary foci (Fig. 10.24).

Retrocardiac space-occupying masses are first visualized on *lateral radiographs* (Fig. 10.25).

Conventional tomograms are rarely obtained. Usually, their purpose is to stratify specific portions of the lung into layers, especially the apex of the lung, when looking for cavities (Fig. 10.26).

Before the investigator decides in favor of invasive diagnostic procedures, an attempt should be made to distinguish between benign and malignant changes. *Computed tomography* offers specific criteria for this purpose (Leung et al. 1990; Heindel 1998; Arenas-Jiménez et al. 2000; Table 10.1).

Table 10.1. Computed tomography criteria for benign and malignant foci

Benign foci	Malignant foci
Smooth contour (Fig. 10.27)	Multiple foci
Calcifications	Central space-occupying mass
Constant size > 2 years	Mediastinal lymphomas
Unremarkable pleura	Pleural findings raising suspicion of disease (Figs. 10.10, 10.11)
Ramifications in 70 % of chronic inflammations (Fig. 10.19)	Ramifications in 95 % in cases of primary bronchial carcinoma
–	Invasive growth beyond the organ

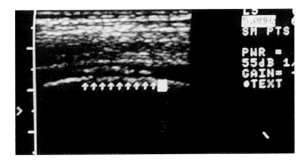

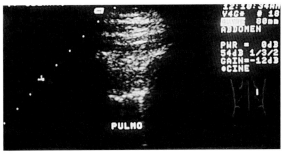

Fig. 10.20. Asbestos plaque (*arrows*) in a callused and thickened pleura

Fig. 10.21. Finely grained uneven surface of the lung in the presence of diffuse lung disease

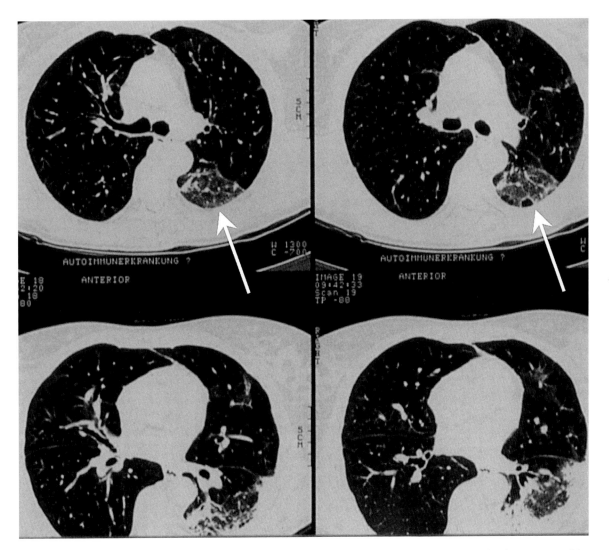

Fig. 10.22. HRCT shows the extent of recent and chronic inflammatory infiltrations in the presence of interstitial pneumonia. In regions of florid disease activity, one finds extensive ground-glass obfuscation of the parenchyma (*arrows*). Here, tissue was obtained by thoracoscopy (histology revealed BOOP, bronchiolitis obliterans with organizing pneumonia)

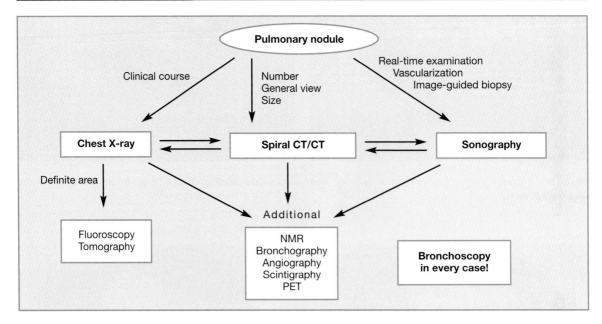

Fig. 10.23. Diagnostic procedure for a circular focus of the lung

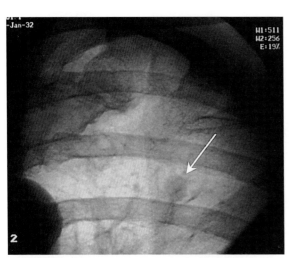

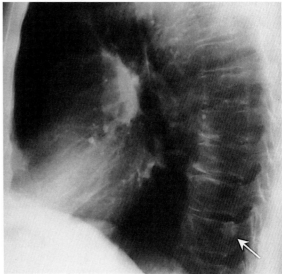

Fig. 10.24. Circular focus in the left upper lobe (*arrow*), demonstrated by fluoroscopy. Removal by thoracoscopy. Histology revealed a tuberculoma

Fig. 10.25. Circular focus (*arrow*) in retrocardiac location, first seen on the lateral radiograph. After removal by thoracoscopy, histology revealed a hamartoma

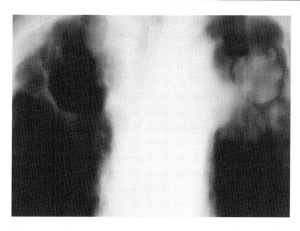

Fig. 10.26. On conventional tomogram, a typical aspergilloma in the left upper lobe

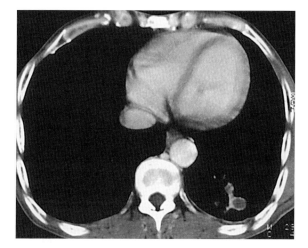

Fig. 10.27. On CT, a focus with smooth margins, a narrow wall, and central hypodense areas in the left upper lobe. *Echinococcus cysticus* was diagnosed from resected tissue

As a rule, *sonography* is used in a targeted fashion with knowledge of other radiographic findings, for the purpose of:

- Preoperative staging:
  - Size of the finding
  - Relationship to the pleura (Fig. 10.28)
  - Invasion into adjacent structures (Figs. 10.3, 10.8)
- Evaluation of vascularization (Fig. 10.28)
- Biopsy under visual control

Bronchoscopy is indispensable to evaluate the central bronchial system.

PET is also an option, as it offers the possibility to distinguish between metabolically inactive fibrosis and a metabolically active malignancy. In this setting, PET will help the clinician to decide whether the indication for surgery should be established (Dewan 1997). However, we observed that active marking does not occur in all cases of malignant circular foci, especially bronchial carcinomas. Thus, they might escape detection on PET.

10.6
Bronchial Carcinoma

Diagnostic procedures for bronchial carcinoma require combined application of all imaging procedures (Yang et al. 1990; Wernecke et al. 1991; Schüder et al. 1991; Yuan et al. 1992; Suzuki et al. 1993; Goldstraw 1995; Pedersen et al. 1996; Sheth et al. 1998; Fritscher-Ravens et al. 1999; Mason et al. 1999; Ukena et al. 2000; Figs. 10.29, 10.30).

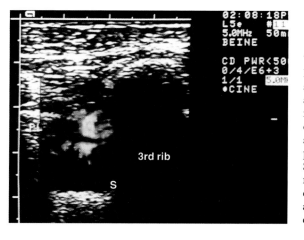

◀

Fig. 10.28. In the left upper lobe, a hypoechoic focus on sonography, that appears to invade the chest wall with a strongly vascularized branch. Sonographic puncture revealed a poorly differentiated adenocarcinoma. A peripheral adenocarcinoma in the upper lobe was confirmed by surgery, in addition to a cord-like callus along the parietal pleura (*PL*). The tumor has not invaded the parietal pleura. Strongly vascularized cord-like pleural calluses or scars may be residues of inflammation. The condition is considered to favor local carcinoma. Unequivocal evidence for an association, however, is currently not available. *S*, space-occupying mass

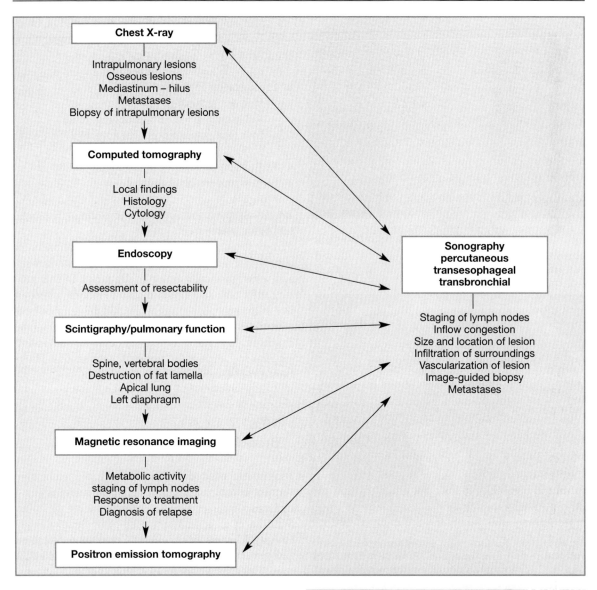

Fig. 10.29. Diagnostic imaging for bronchial carcinoma

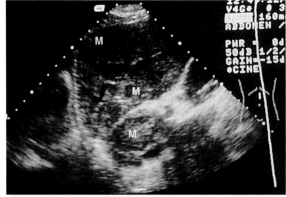

Fig. 10.30. Multiple, rather hypoechoic metastases (*M*) on the sonographic longitudinal section through the left lobe of the liver and the caudate lobe

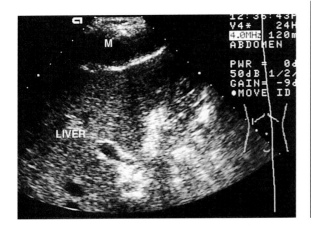

Fig. 10.31. On the sonographic flank section in the right side, rather hypoechoic metastasis (*M*) with smooth margins, cranial to the liver, in the diaphragm of a patient with known metastatic renal cell carcinoma

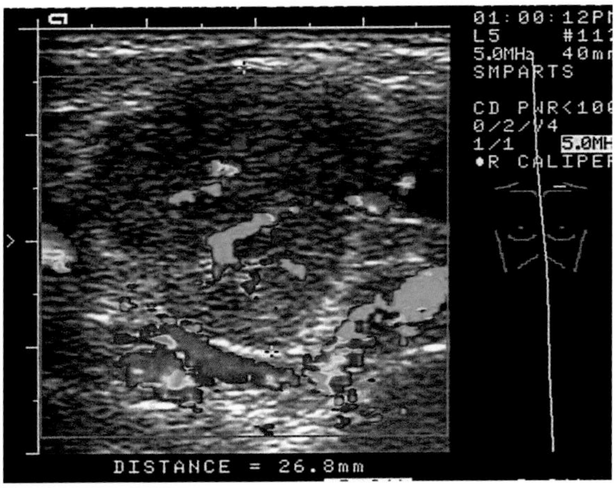

Fig. 10.32. Left side, supraclavicular, strongly vascularized lymph node metastasis. Radiographs showed tumor formation in the upper anterior mediastinum, extending up to the left hilum. Sonographic puncture: tumor cells of a small-cell anaplastic carcinoma

10.7
Search for Metastases in the Lung and Pleura

Survey radiographs are the basic procedure, complemented by sonography in all accessible regions (Figs. 10.30–10.32).
Spiral CT provides the best overview of the entire lung parenchyma (Munden et al. 1997; Heindel 1998, Tuengerthal 1998). *Bronchoscopy* is used to evaluate the central respiratory tract and to obtain material for histological and cytological investigation.
PET is sufficiently sensitive (Reske et al. 1996; Knopp and Bischoff 1998) in cases of:

- Differentiated thyroid carcinoma (iodine-accumulating recurrent disease)
- Local recurrence and lymph node staging in cases of non-small cell bronchial carcinoma
- Colorectal carcinoma with enhanced tumor marker activity
- Malignant melanoma (stage II and III)
- Malignant lymphoma

Acknowledgments. We thank Assistant Professor R. Loose, Head of the Institute for Diagnostic and Interventional Radiology at the North Nuremberg Clinic, for providing us with radiological findings.

References

Agrons GA, Rosado-de-Christenson ML, Kirejczyk WM et al. (1998) Pulmonary inflammatory pseudotumor: radiologic features. Radiology 206:511–518

Arcasoy SM, Jett JR (1997) Current concepts: superior pulmonary sulcus tumors and Pancoast's syndrome. New Engl J Med 337:1370–1376

Arenas-Jiménez J, Alonso-Charterina S, Sánchez-Payá J et al. (2000) Evaluation of CT findings for diagnosis of pleural effusions. Eur Radiol 10:681–690

Deutsche Gesellschaft für Pneumologie (1994) Empfehlungen zur Diagnostik und Therapie von Lungenkrankheiten. Pneumologie 48:281–286

Dewan NA (1997) Likelihood of malignancy in a solitary pulmonary nodule. Comparison of Bayesian analysis and results of FDG-PET scan. Chest 112:416–422

Dubs-Kunz B (1996) Sonography of the chest wall. Eur J Ultrasound 3:102–111

Düster P, Mayer E, Kramm T et al. (2000) Solitäre fibröse Pleuratumoren – Seltene Tumoren mit unvorhersehbarem klinischen Verhalten. Pneumologie 54:16–19

Fraser RS, Colman N, Müller NL, Paré PD (1999a) Diagnosis of Diseases of the Chest. Saunders, Philadelphia, S 563–594

Fraser RS, Colman N, Müller NL, Paré PD (1999b) Diagnosis of diseases of the chest. Saunders, London, S 2807–2847

Fritscher-Ravens A, Petrasch S, Reinacher-Schick A et al. (1999) Diagnostic value of endoscopic ultrasonography-guided fine-needle aspiration cytology of mediastinal masses in patients with intrapulmonary lesions and nondiagnostic bronchoscopy. Respiration 66:150–155

Goldstraw P (1995) Mediastinal disorders. Mediastinal masses. In: Brewis RAL, Corrin B, Geddes DM, Gibson GJ (eds) Respiratory medicine. Saunders, London, S 1582

Heindel W (1998) Lungentumoren. In: Krahe T (Hrsg) Bildgebende Diagnostik von Lunge und Pleura. Thieme, Stuttgart, S 217–264

Knopp MV, Bischoff H (1998) Positronenemissionstomographie. In: Drings P, Vogt-Moykopf I (Hrsg) Thoraxtumoren. Springer, Berlin Heidelberg New York Tokyo, S 191–201

Layer G, Schmitteckert H, Steudel A et al. (1999) MRT, CT und Sonographie in der präoperativen Beurteilung der Primärtumorausdehnung beim malignen Pleuramesotheliom. Fortschr Röntgenstr 170:365–370

Leung AN, Müller NL, Miller RR (1990) CT in differential diagnosis of diffuse pleural disease. AJR 154:487–492

Loddenkemper R, Boutin C (1993) Thoracoscopy: present diagnostic and therapeutic indications. Eur Respir J 6:1544–1555

Mason AC, Miller BH, Krasna MJ et al. (1999) Accuracy of CT for the detection of pleural adhesions. Chest 115:423–427

Mathis G (1997a) Thoraxsonography-Part I: Chest wall and pleura. Ultrasound Med Biol 23:1131–1139

Mathis G (1997b) Thoraxsonography-Part II: Peripheral pulmonary consolidation. Ultrasound Med Biol 23:1141–1153

Morris V, Wiggins J (1992) Current management of pleural disease. Brit J Hosp Med 47:753–758

Munden RF, Pugatch RD, Liptay MJ et al. (1997) Small pulmonary lesions detected at CT: clinical importance. Radiology 202:105–110

Padovani B, Mouroux J, Seksik L et al. (1993) Chest wall invasion by bronchogenic carcinoma: evaluation with MR imaging. Radiology 187:33–38

Pedersen BH, Vilmann P, Folke K et al. (1996) Endoscopic ultrasonography and real-time guided fine-needle aspiration biopsy of solid lesions of the mediastinum suspected of malignancy. Chest 110:539–544

Rapoport S, Blair DN, McCarthy SM et al. (1988) Brachial plexus: Correlation of MR imaging with CT and pathologic findings. Radiology 167:161–165

Remy-Jardin M, Remy J, Giraud F et al. (1993) Pulmonary nodules: Detection with thick-section spiral CT versus conventional CT. Radiology 187:513–520

Reske SN, Bares R, Büll U et al. (1996) Klinische Wertigkeit der Positronen-Emissions-Tomographie (PET) bei onkologischen Fragestellungen: Ergebnisse einer interdisziplinären Konsensuskonferenz. Nucl Med 35:42–52

Reynolds HY (1998) Diagnostic and management strategies for diffuse interstitial lung disease. Chest 113:192–202

Rozenshtein A, White CS, Austin JHM et al. (1998) Incidental lung carcinoma detected at CT in patients selected for lung volume reduction surgery to treat severe pulmonary emphysema. Radiology 207:487–490

Schüder G, Isringhaus H, Kubale B et al. (1991) Endoscopic ultrasonography of the mediastinum in the diagnosis of bronchial carcinoma. Thorac Cardiovasc Surg 39:299–303

Sheth S, Hamper UM, Stanley DB et al. (1999) US guidance for thoracic biopsy: a valuable alternative to CT. Radiology 210:721–726

Suzuki N, Saitoh T, Kitamura S et al. (1993) Tumor invasion of the chest wall in lung cancer: diagnosis with US. Radiology 187:39–42

Swensen SJ, Aughenbaugh GL, Myers JL et al. (1997) Diffuse lung disease: Diagnostic accuracy of CT in patients undergoing surgical biopsy of the lung. Radiology 205:229–234

Tuengerthal SJ (1998) Diagnostik der Lungenmetastasen. In: Drings P, Vogt-Moykopf I (Hrsg) Thoraxtumoren. Springer, Berlin Heidelberg New York Tokyo, S 615–639

Ukena D, Hellwig D, Palm I et al. (2000) Stellenwert der Positronen-Emissions-Tomographie mit 18-Fluor-Desoxyglukose (FDG-PET) in der Rezidivdiagnostik des Bronchialkarzinoms. Pneumologie 54:49–53

Vahlensieck M (1998) Interstitielle Lungenerkrankungen. In: Krahe T (Hrsg) Bildgebende Diagnostik von Lunge und Pleura. Thieme, Stuttgart, S 127–155

Wernecke K, Vassallo P, Hoffmann G et al. (1991) Value of sonography in monitoring the therapeutic response of mediastinal lymphoma: comparison with chest radiography and CT. AJR 165:265–272

Yang PC, Luh KT, Wu HD et al. (1990) Lung tumors associated with obstructive pneumonitis: US studies. Radiology 174:717–720

Yuan A, Yang PC, Chang DB et al. (1992) Ultrasound-guided aspiration biopsy of small peripheral pulmonary nodules. Chest 101:926–930

Subject Index

abdominal trauma 31
abscess 37, 41, 157
– drainage 43, 158
– chest wall abscess 7, 8
– lung abscess 37, 41, 157, 158, 167
absorption 137, 138
acoustic shadow 1, 137, 141
actinomycosis 53
air 138
air bronchogram 37, 39, 73, 125, 128, 129, 167
aliasing 144
anatomy, sonographic 91 ff., 114
aorta 122, 159
aortico-pulmonary window 86, 91, 117
arcuate artifact 140
artifacts 137 ff.
asbestosis 27, 170
aspergilloma 54, 173
aspiration cytology 151
atelectasis 23, 72 ff., 125
attenuation 137
autofluorescence 114

background noise 143
bacteriological investigation 81
biopsy see also puncture 28, 54, 55, 88, 147 ff., 172
blood coagulum 160
bone 138
breathing difficulties 24
bronchial aerogram 39
bronchial anatomy 114
bronchial carcinoma 50 ff., 107, 148, 153, 168, 173
bronchial obstruction 39
bronchial reflex, central 58
bronchiolitis obliterans 171
bronchopneumogram 39
bronchoscopy 167

calcification 25, 29
carcinoid 100

carcinoma 50 ff., 65, 173
– adenocarcinoma 51 ff., 166, 173
– adenoid-cystic 165
– anaplastic 175
– bronchoalveolar 55
– diagnostic imaging 174
– large-cell 51
– renal cell carcinoma 175
– squamous cell carcinoma 51 ff.
– thyroid carcinoma 175
cardiac wall, infiltration 28
catheter 131, 152
chest pain 163
chest wall 3 f., 7 ff.
– infiltration, invasion 15, 29, 52
chest X-ray
– circular focus 170
– fluoroscopy 170
– lung carcinoma 50
– mediastinum 97
– pleural effusions 20
– pleuritis 22
– pneumonia 42
– pneumothorax 30
– pulmonary embolism 66
– tuberculosis 44
"chimney" phenomenon 13
chondroma 25
chronic obstructive lung disease 31
circular focus 133, 170 ff.
circulation 41, 65, 78, 144
colliquation 41, 45, 54, 134
color-Doppler sign 19, 29
color Doppler sonography
– artifacts 143 f.
– atelectasis 73, 75, 81, 125, 133
– carcinoma 50 ff., 175
– hematoma 121
– leg veins 68
– mediastinum 97 f.
– needle 98, 153
– osteolysis 14 f.
– pleural effusion 19
– pleuritis 24
– pneumonia 41, 168
– pneumonia, poststenotic 39

– pulmonary artery 81, 144
– pulmonary artery, thrombosis 87
– pulmonary embolism 65, 68
– pulmonary vein 81, 144
– puncture 98, 148 f.
– rib 14 f.
– white hemithorax 121, 125, 133
comet-tail artifact 17, 139, 142
compression atelectasis 65, 72 ff., 129
computed tomography 163 ff.
– abscess drainage 41
– atelectasis 80 ff.
– diaphragmatic lipoma 32
– mediastinum 97
– mesothelioma 28 f.
– neoplasm 50
– pneumonia 40, 167
– pulmonary embolism 67
– puncture 148
– stepwise diagnostic procedures 163 ff.
– white hemithorax 122 ff.
consistency of the surfaces 138
consolidation 37, 50
contour 50
contraindications 104, 147
contusion, lung 89
cortical reflex 12 ff.
cyst, mediastinal 100

deep vein thrombosis 68
detection of pathogens 42
device settings 3
diagnostic imaging 164, 174
diagnostic procedure 172
diaphragm 31 ff., 138
– diaphragmatic crura 31
– diaphragmatic fold 34
– diaphragmatic hernia 31
– diaphragmatic lipoma 32
– diaphragmatic paralysis 33
– metastasis on the diaphragm 31 f.
– rupture of the diaphragm 31

diffraction 137, 141
dilatation heart 69
dilatation, mechanical 117
directional artifact 143
dispersion 137
drainage 74, 142, 156 ff.
- catheter 131, 152
- lung abscess 158
dysphagia 101
dyspnea 65

echinococcus cysticus 47
echocardiography 69
echo enhancement 141
echo obliteration 138, 141
echo resolution artifact 141
echo transmission 15
embolism, see also pulmonary
    embolism 57 ff.
emergency examination 13, 30
empyema 22, 24, 122
endoscopic ultrasound 3
- endobronchial 113 ff.
- transesophageal 104 ff.
endosonography 107 ff.
esophageal carcinoma 101 f.
esophageal disease 101, 117
examination 4 f., 94 ff.
exsudate 21

farmer's lung 48
fatty liver 33
fibrolipoma 8, 165
fibrothorax 128
filter 143
fine needle aspiration, see also
    puncture 104, 157
fluid alveogram 37
fluid bronchogram 39, 82, 125,
    132
fluid-color sign 19, 157
flow profiles 78
follow-up 15, 19, 43

germ cell carcinoma 100

hamartoma 55
hemangiofibroma 55
hematoma 7, 121
hematopericardium 101
hemithorax, white 28
hemoptysis 159
hemorrhages 57
hemothorax 22
hiatal hernia, axial 31
histiocytoma 55
hyalinosis 51

implications, clinical 106
indications 1, 97, 163 ff.
- pneumonia 42
infarction pneumonia 65
infiltration, vessels 98
initial lung echo 139
interstitial lung disease 48, 171 ff.
interventional chest sonography 147
- pneumonia 42
- mediastinum, transesophageal
    104
- mediastinum, transthoracic 97
invasive sonography 2
investigation procedure 3, 91

laser therapy 115
leiomyoma 117
leukemia, chronic lymphatic 101
"lighthouse" phenomenon 13
lipoma 7, 8, 25 f., 32, 165 f., 170
lobar pneumonia 38, 130
lung abscess 41 f., 135, 158
lung carcinoma see also bronchial
    carcinoma 50 ff.
lung consolidation 37 ff., 156
- congenital 90
- inflammmatory 37 ff.
- mechanical 72 ff.
- neoplastic 50 ff.
- transbronchial 116
- vascular 57 ff.
lung contusion 13, 89
lung opacity 119
lymph node 7 ff.
- inflammatory 10 ff.
- malignant lymphoma 11, 98
- mediastinal 104 ff.
- metastases 10 f., 50, 99
- parabronchial 113
- technique 3
- tuberculosis 98
lymphoma, malignant 9 ff., 159, 175

magnetic resonance tomography
- indication 167
- lung carcinoma 50
- mesothelioma 28
- Pancoast tumor 164
- pneumonia 167
margin, sharp 37, 50
marginal shadows 138, 141
mediastinoscopy 107
mediastinum 91 ff.
- cyst 100
- lymph node 104 ff.
- masses 116
- thymoma 99
- transbronchial 116
- transesophageal 104 ff.

- transthoracic 91 ff.
- tumor 159
melanoma 175
mesothelioma 27 ff., 152, 159, 165 f.
metastases 14
- chest wall 15
- diaphragm 31
- lung 54, 175
- mediastinum 98
- pleural 25 f., 120
- rib 14
microabscess 41, 80
miliary tuberculosis 44, 45
mirror artifacts 139 ff.
monitoring 15
- pneumonia 43
motion artifact 144

necrosis 54, 134
neonatology 32
neovascularization 15, 50
neuroendocrine tumor 126
newborn babies 31 f.
noise 141
non-Hodgkin's lymphoma 9, 12, 97,
    124, 148, 159

obstruction, bronchial 39
obstructive atelectasis 76 ff.
osteolysis 14
overall enhancement 143

Pancoast tumor 14, 163
panoramic image 3, 99
paralysis, diaphragm 33
parathyroid 100
pathogen detection 42
pericardial effusion 99, 101
pericardium, invasion, infiltration 29,
    99
physics 137
pitfalls 137
plasma cell tumor 15
pleura, adherent 34, 73
- callus 173
- carcinosis 26, 124, 165
- fragmentation 45, 48
- normal 17
- plaque 28
- tumors 8, 25 f.
pleural effusion 18 ff., 60, 120 ff.,
    165
- carcinomatosis 26, 120, 124, 165
- cavities 23, 24, 123
- estimation of the volume 20
- focal 22, 44
- measure 20
- minimal 45, 48
- septation 24

pleural empyema 24 f., 122, 165
– fistula 24
– drainage 152, 156
pleural fibrosis 29 f.
pleural forceps biopsy 155
pleural mesothelioma 25, 27 ff., 152
– diaphragm infiltration 31
pleural metastases 25 ff.
pleural shifting 25
pleural solid changes 22
pleuritis 22 ff., 165
pleurodesis 165
pleuropneumonia 167
pneumonia 37 ff., 65, 167
– bronchopneumonia 39
– engorgement phase 37
– focal pneumonia 37
– interstitial 48, 171
– lobar 38
– poststenotic 39, 41
– segmental pneumonia 40
– viral pneumonia 38
pneumothorax 29 f., 154, 159 f.
positron emisson tomography (PET)
   167, 174
probe 3 ff.
pulmonary abscess 24
pulmonary angiography 67
pulmonary artery 78, 81, 86, 144
pulmonary blastoma 127
pulmonary embolism 57 ff.
pulmonary infarction 57 ff.
– early pulmonary infarction 58
– late pulmonary infarction 58
– infarction pneumonia 61
pulmonary nodule 172
pulmonary sequestration 90
pulmonary vein 78, 81, 86, 144
pulse repetition frequency 143
puncture 81
– artifacts 143
– catheter 131
– chest wall 15
– circular focus 170
– empyema 25
– esophageal carcinoma 102
– interventional sonography 147 ff.
– lung carcinoma 157
– mediastinal cyst 100
– mediastinal lymph node metastasis
   98
– mediastinum 157
– mesothelioma 28, 165
– methods 149
– miliary tuberculosis 45
– needle 150 f.
– needle artifact 143
– osteolysis 14
– pleural carcinosis 120

– pleural empyema 24
– transbronchial 114, 116
– transesophageal 104 ff.

ramification 50
real-time examination 33, 104, 144
reflection 137
refraction 137
repetitive echo 138 f.
resonance artifact 142
respiratory movement 25
reventilation 73
reverberation 29, 37, 137 ff.
rib fracture 12 f., 163 f.
rib metastasis 14
right heart thrombus 69
right heart tumor 101
ring-down artifact 143
roughness 138

scatter lens artifact 141 f.
schwannoma 25
scintigraphy 66, 115, 174
septation 24, 165
sequestration, pulmonary 90
shadow, acoustic 1, 137 f., 141
shortening phenomenon 141 f.
signal embolism 60
slice thickness 142
slice thickness artifact 142
soft tissue tumor 9, 154
sonic shadow areas 1
sonomorphology
– atelectasis 72
– carcinoma 50
– compression atelectasis 72
– lymph nodes 9
– metastases 55
– obstructive atelectasis 80
– pleuritis 22
– pneumonia 37
– pulmonary infarction 58
– thymoma 100
– tuberculosis 45
source of embolism 67 f.
source of error 137
space-occupying mass
– predominantly liquid 119 ff.
– predominantly solid 125 ff.
splenic enlargement 33
split pleura 24 f.
staging
– endobronchial 115
– mediastinal 106
stent 117
stepwise diagnostic imaging 163 ff.
sternum fracture 12 ff.

subclavian artery stenosis 144
subclavian vein thrombosis 53
subclavian vessels 14
symptoms 1

technical equipment, requirements 3,
   104, 113, 148
– thoracentesis 154 f.
– trocar technique 152
therapy
– endobronchial 117
thoracocentesis 21, 154 f.
thoracoscopy 52, 104, 155, 167
– video-assisted 52, 155
thoracotomy 107
thorax trauma 13, 29, 89
thorax wall see also chest wall
– infiltration 15, 28
– metastasis 154
– trauma 13, 29
thrombosis
– leg vein 68
– pulmonary artery 87
– subclavian vein 53
– transbronchial 116
– vena cava 97
thrombus, intracardial 69
thymoma 100, 159
thyroid 98, 100
Tietze's syndrome 2
time-motion 33
tomogram 170
transbronchial sonography 2, 113
transducer 3 f.
transesophageal sonography 104
transhepatic examination 5
transudate 21
tuberculosis 44 ff.
– abscess, cold 8
– lymph nodes 98
– miliary tuberculosis 44 f.
– pleurisy 23
– tuberculoma 46
tumor
– benign pleural 25
– formation 83
– mediastinum 96
– staging 52, 115

vaccine metastases 159
vascular signs 60
vascularization 9, 15, 50, 53, 174
vessel neoformation 14
vibration artifact 144
viral pneumonia 38

white hemithorax 119 ff.